The Objective Structured Clinical Examination

Brian Hodges

The Objective Structured Clinical Examination

A Socio-History

LAP LAMBERT Academic Publishing

Impressum/Imprint (nur für Deutschland/ only for Germany)
Bibliografische Information der Deutschen Nationalbibliothek: Die Deutsche Nationalbibliothek verzeichnet diese Publikation in der Deutschen Nationalbibliografie; detaillierte bibliografische Daten sind im Internet über http://dnb.d-nb.de abrufbar.
Alle in diesem Buch genannten Marken und Produktnamen unterliegen warenzeichen-, marken- oder patentrechtlichem Schutz bzw. sind Warenzeichen oder eingetragene Warenzeichen der jeweiligen Inhaber. Die Wiedergabe von Marken, Produktnamen, Gebrauchsnamen, Handelsnamen, Warenbezeichnungen u.s.w. in diesem Werk berechtigt auch ohne besondere Kennzeichnung nicht zu der Annahme, dass solche Namen im Sinne der Warenzeichen- und Markenschutzgesetzgebung als frei zu betrachten wären und daher von jedermann benutzt werden dürften.

Coverbild: www.purestockx.com

Verlag: LAP LAMBERT Academic Publishing AG & Co. KG
Theodor-Heuss-Ring 26, 50668 Köln, Germany
Telefon: +49 681 3720-310, Telefax: +49 681 3720-3109, Email: info@lap-publishing.com

Herstellung in Deutschland:
Schaltungsdienst Lange o.H.G., Berlin
Books on Demand GmbH, Norderstedt
Reha GmbH, Saarbrücken
Amazon Distribution GmbH, Leipzig
ISBN: 978-3-8383-0181-5

Imprint (only for USA, GB)
Bibliographic information published by the Deutsche Nationalbibliothek: The Deutsche Nationalbibliothek lists this publication in the Deutsche Nationalbibliografie; detailed bibliographic data are available in the Internet at http://dnb.d-nb.de.
Any brand names and product names mentioned in this book are subject to trademark, brand or patent protection and are trademarks or registered trademarks of their respective holders. The use of brand names, product names, common names, trade names, product descriptions etc. even without a particular marking in this works is in no way to be construed to mean that such names may be regarded as unrestricted in respect of trademark and brand protection legislation and could thus be used by anyone.

Cover image: www.purestockx.com

Publisher:
LAP LAMBERT Academic Publishing AG & Co. KG
Theodor-Heuss-Ring 26, 50668 Köln, Germany
Phone: +49 681 3720-310, Fax: +49 681 3720-3109, Email: info@lap-publishing.com

THE OBJECTIVE STRUCTURED CLINICAL EXAMINATION:

A SOCIO-HISTORICAL STUDY

For Hobbes

CHAPTER 1: RETHINKING THE HISTORY OF THE OSCE

As for what motivated me, it is quite simple.... It was curiosity, the only kind of
curiosity, in any case, that is worth acting upon with a degree of obstinacy; not the
curiosity that seeks to assimilate what it is proper for one to know, but that which
enables one to get free of oneself.... There are times in life when the question of
knowing if one can think differently than one sees, is absolutely necessary if one is to
go on looking and reflecting at all (Foucault 1976/1990, pp. 8-9).

1.1   Introduction

In 1975, a Scottish professor of medicine named Ronald Harden invented a new form
of examination called the Objective Structured Clinical Examination (OSCE) for the
assessment of medical students at the University of Dundee (Harden, Stevenson,
Downie & Wilson, 1979). Although medical student examinations had emphasized
observed interactions with patients since the early twentieth century, this OSCE
examination was radically different from anything that had been utilized before. First,
during the OSCE examination, students were observed interacting with not just one
patient -- but with a whole series. The examination involved several dozen clinical
interactions, each completed in a fixed amount of time, evaluated with standard
measurement instruments and following a strict rotation schedule though a set of
adjacent rooms, as shown in Figure 1. In each room an examiner observed and rated
student performance. Some of the patients interviewed and examined by students
were "simulated patients", a technique of using actors and actresses to portray the
problems presented by patients that was developed by Howard Barrows in California
in the 1960s (Barrows & Abrahamson, 1964; Barrows, 1971). Assessment with
OSCEs and simulated patients represented a totally new direction in examination of
competence that emphasized 'standardization' and 'objectivity'.[1]

---

[1] Throughout this thesis, I have used single quotation marks to problematize a word or
discourse.

Figure 1: Students Waiting for the Bell to Begin an OSCE

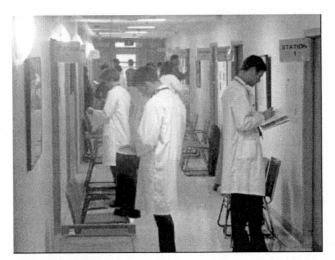

(Photo provided by Diana Tabak)

Figure 2: Bird's Eye View of the Layout of an OSCE

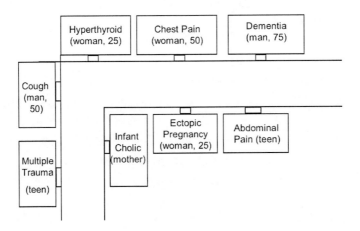

6

In the two decades that followed, OSCE-type, multiple-station examinations enjoyed an extraordinary success, not only in the UK, but across the world. In the 1980s, they were widely adopted by medical schools in the United Kingdom, Holland, the United States and Canada. In the 1990s, they were taken up as the main format of assessment for national medical licensure in Canada, then as a mandatory examination for all international medical gradates wishing to train in the United States, and finally, in 2005, for all American medical graduates. In Canada, over 2000 individuals are marshalled to participate in the national OSCE held in 14 Canadian cites annually. In the United States, the need to process a large number of candidates led to the establishment of five dedicated "testing centres" that run the largest multi-station, simulated patient examination in history. Since 2005, these American testing centres have examined over 25,000 medical graduates each year. Meanwhile, most North American health professions other than medicine have also adopted OSCEs and their variations for training and licensure. In Canada, for example, there are OSCEs for midwives, nurses, pharmacists, physiotherapists and massage therapists. In the UK, an OSCE has become the only route to promotion for police officers, and the United Nations is said to be adopting OSCEs for the training and assessment of peacekeepers! OSCEs are rapidly being adopted in many countries of Asia, South America and Africa and China has announced a large project to develop 'modern assessment methods' that include OSCEs in order to 'meet international standards'.

What is going on? Why has this relatively simple examination spread so quickly into every aspect of education and assessment, not only in medicine, or even just health professions, but education of all sorts? What has been behind the rapid and enthusiastic adoption of this method of assessment in European and North American countries, as well as on the Asian and African continents? In order to answer these questions, it is necessary to address two issues. First, what is the nature and of function of any examination? That is, what are the historical, political and sociological functions of examinations? Second, why *this* examination? What are the contingencies that favoured the emergence and widespread adoption of this multi-station, simulated patient-based examination at this particular time in history?

Examinations are ubiquitous in the lives of human beings. Within the first minutes of life, the newborn is 'examined' for deviations from the norm. Regular examinations are a part of school life between kindergarten and high school graduation, and later as the portal to higher education. University and college life are dominated by examinations. Then there are the examinations to get a job, to ascertain health status for insurance and for leisure activities such as scuba diving or swimming. Even popular magazines are full of self-administered tests that we willing use on ourselves to assess everything from body shape to sexual responsiveness.

In Euro-American countries, we examine and are examined continually. It is remarkable that so little has been written about this phenomenon of continuous examination. While myriad books and articles explore *how* to conduct examinations, evaluations and assessments, there has been very little exploration of all this examination from a sociological perspective. However, Michel Foucault claimed that examinations are among the most important, yet least studied, of the Post-Enlightenment techniques for modifying and controlling human behaviour:

The superimposition of power relations and knowledge relations assumes in the examination all its visible brilliance. It is yet another innovation of the classical age that the historians of science have left unexplored.... Who will write the more general, more fluid, but also more determinant history of the 'examination' – its rituals, its methods, it character and their roles, its play of questions and answers, it systems of marking and classification? (Foucault, 1975/1995, pp. 184-5)

A particularly fertile ground for studying the power of examinations is the domain of health professional education where examinations are found across the continuum of professional education and practice. Professional lives start with competitive selection examinations that control entry to prestigious and potentially lucrative careers; continue with in-training examinations that regularly punctuate professional education; pass through an intensive phase of professional certification and licensure testing; and trickle off into a continuous series of evaluations that comprise 'maintenance of competence' and 'recertification'.

Although there are variations around the world, most medical schools today provide two to four years of theoretical education prior to introducing clinical rotations in hospitals and offices. The final two years in most medical schools are comprised of a set of practical rotations called the "clinical clerkship" that is designed to prepare

8

students for another long practical apprenticeship called the "residency". This period of two to five years follows medical school and is designed to allow students to consolidate and apply their knowledge and skills in clinical settings of family medicine or a medical specialty. These large blocks of practical training have always had a great emphasis on performance, and often ended with an examination. What has changed in recent years is the nature of the tools used to assess that performance.

Going back to early medical guilds, assessment of doctors in training has long involved evaluation by supervisors. In the nineteenth century, formal written tests of knowledge were developed in many medical schools. During the twentieth century, countries developed national certification examinations at the end of medical training. These consisted of written tests of knowledge and in some cases "oral examinations" with performance elements. The performance elements tested were quite variable, ranging from the ability of students to "think on their feet" in front of examinations panels, to more formal observations of their skills in interviewing and examination patients. However, oral examinations were highly variable in their structure and their content and standards for performance were left to the physician examiners. In the mid-twentieth century, particularly in the US, UK and Canada, dissatisfaction with a perceived over-emphasis on competence-as-written knowledge led to the development of examinations that included much more structured observation of 'performance'.

1.2   The Birth of the OSCE
In the second half of the twentieth century, health professional assessment was influenced by an influx of professional educators and psychometricians who brought with them the perspectives of testing theory, measurement and statistics. Concepts such as reliability and validity, which were not previously very prominent in the design and administration of performance-based tests, began to alter the way health professional educators thought about what were good methods of assessment. In particular, attention to reliability, or the degree to which testing instruments yield the same score on different occasions or with different observers, meant that examinations were pushed in the direction of multiple observers and multiple scenarios.

A number of authors recount this history and critique the use of oral examinations (Abrahamson, 1985; Davidson, 1983; Muzzin & Hart, 1985; Jayawickramarajah, 1985; Valberg & Stuart 1983). The research of Christine McGuire (1966), one of the first non-physician medical educators to show that oral examinations were inadequate, is often cited. McGuire, herself the subject of a short history (Harris & Simpson, 2005), is most often credited with 'killing' oral examinations. In a key study conducted for the National Board of Medical Examiners in the United States, she showed that for 10,000 US medical student oral examinations, the average correlation between examiner scores was less than 0.25. This led to the discontinuation of oral examination of US medical students in 1963 (McGuire, 1966).

Many books and articles report that during the 1960s and 1970s, there was great interest in the UK, Canada and the USA in creating new forms of performance-based examinations that would be designed to increase the consistency of examiner judgments (e.g. Dauphinee, 2004; Miller, 1990; Wallace, 1997). This could be achieved in two ways: by increasing the number of independent observations and by standardizing examination materials. Until the 1960s, clinical testing rested on the demonstration of performance on 'real' hospitalized or clinic patients. The major change that occurred in the 1960s was the development of methods to simulate or standardize teaching and testing cases. Several developments occurred in a short period of time, including Howard Barrows' use of actors trained to present histories and physical findings to students (Barrows & Abramson, 1964), Paula Stillman's coaching of patients and their family members to teach and assess students (Stillman, Sabers & Redfield, 1976; 1977), and the introduction into the classroom of women called "gynaecological teaching associates", who used their own bodies to demonstrate pelvic examination techniques (Livingstone & Ostrow, 1978).

According to Wallace (1997), all of these inventions were renamed "standardized patients" after about 1980 at a time when the key advantages of their use were believed to be reproducible performances, easy control of content, tolerance of multiple performances, and undetectability (Sanson-Fisher & Poole, 1980; Owen & Winkler, 1974; Norman, Neufeld, Walsh, Woodward & McConvey, 1985). As a result, health professional schools around the world developed standardized patient programs.

While all of the developments described above led to the standardization of teaching and assessment in medicine, they did not address the perceived need for multiple observations during examinations. This element was finally dealt with in 1975 with the invention of the Objective Structured Clinical Examination (OSCE). Several publications specifically recount the history of the OSCE (for example: Wallace, 1997; Rothman & Cohen, 1995; Nayer, 1993; Howley, 2004). First described by Harden and Gleason in 1975, an OSCE was a timed examination in which students moved through a series of scenarios or stations, in each of which they performed a standardized task, often involving interaction with a patient, or with other types of models or simulations (Harden & Gleason, 1979). Students were observed demonstrating some combination of history-taking, physical examination or other clinical skills. In each station, candidates' performances were rated on standardized rating scales. After 1979, OSCEs spread rapidly and became the subject of hundreds of articles in medical education generally (Rothman & Cohen, 1995; Kowlovitz, Hoole & Sloane, 1991; Nayer, 1993) and in specialty areas such as paediatrics (Matsell, Wolfish & Hsu, 1991), surgery (Sloan, Donnelly, Johnson, Swartz & Strodel, 1993), obstetrics and gynaecology (McFaul, Taylor & Howie, 1993) and psychiatry (Hodges, Regehr, Hanson & McNaughton, 1997).

In health professions other than medicine, there was also an asymptotic growth of the use of OSCE-type examinations. This included pharmacy (Sibbald & Regehr, 2003), physiotherapy (Nayer, 1993), massage therapy (College of Massage Therapists, 2005), nursing (Major, 2005), midwifery (Govaerts, van der Vleuten & Schuwirth, 2002), dentistry (Manogue & Brown, 1998) and veterinary medicine (Bark & Cohen, 2002). Each of the articles in specialty medicine and in the various other health professions has recounted a history of continuous progress and refinement in the assessment using OSCEs.

The OSCE came to Canada as a result of the efforts of Ian Hart, an internist who spent a sabbatical with his medical school colleague, Ronald Harden, in Dundee in the early 1980s. Hart implement the OSCE at the University of Ottawa and later

11

promoted it internationally. Dauphinee noted that, in Canada, the OSCE's "value as a formative feedback tool was widely accepted quite rapidly, but its role in assessment took much longer". However, momentum grew and it was finally adopted "in many guises" (Dauphinee, 2004, p. 116). A national licensure OSCE for all medical graduates was adopted in Canada in 1995 (Reznick et al., 1992), and the Education Commission on Foreign Medical Graduates adopted a multi-station, standardized patient-based examination for all international graduates in the US in 1998 (Sutnick et al., 1994, Ben-David et al., 1999). In 2004, a similar examination called the Clinical Skills Assessment (CSA) became a requirement for all medical school graduates in the United States (Dillon, Boulet, Hawkins & Swanson, 2004). By the 1990s, the OSCE and other multi-station, standardized examinations were spreading around the world. As of the early 21st century, most medical schools in North America and Australia/New Zealand used OSCE-type examinations and they were increasingly being adopted in Europe and growing numbers of schools in Africa, South America and Asia (Stern, Friedman Ben-David, Norcini, Wojtczak & Schwarz, 2006).

It is important to note that there have been many terms used in the literature for multiple-station performance-based examinations, such as Clinical Skills Examination (CSX), Clinical Performance Examination (CPX), Clinical Skills Assessment (CSA), Objective Structured Performance Examination (OSPE), Teaching Objective Structured Clinical Examination (TOSCE), Objective Structured Assessments of Technical Skills (OSATS), among others. Although individuals and institutions like to develop and promote their own 'brand' of performance-based assessment examination, most authors, conference planners and health professional educators appear to use the term OSCE as a general term for all multi-station, performance-based examinations. This was illustrated in my search of the Pub-Med data base for the term "OSCE", which yielded 588 articles. Searching the other terms yielded a few dozen articles at most and many searches were confounded because of other medical and scientific entities using the same acronyms. Only the Organization for Security and Cooperation in Europe shares the term OSCE, and this was never cited in the health professional literature. Thus, to be consistent, I have used the term OSCE in this research to represent broadly all multi-station performance-based examinations.

1.3   The Research Problem

Standard medical educators' accounts of the birth of OSCEs and standardized patients presented as self-evident that the small Dundee OSCE of 1975 would inevitably evolve into a huge US licensure examination. Indeed, the literature tends to conceptualize the history of assessment in medicine, the trajectory of performance-based assessment, and the emergence of OSCEs and SPs as one long, unitary sweep.

These "internalist" accounts of OSCE history present the OSCE as a triumph of scientific and statistical advancement in the assessment of medical competence. Such a presentation is congruent with positivism and its orientation toward progress, the unity of knowledge, empiricism and rationalism (Denzin & Lincoln, 2000). Generally adopting an optimistic stance, positivist medical authors place most developments in assessment within the context of medical education's advancement through science and rationality. For example, Wallace wrote in the following way about the twin development of SPs and OSCEs:

In looking back on any human endeavour, it is always interesting to see how diverse are the motivations that shape history. Altruism and egotism entwined create the path, inspire the wisdom that has shaped the movement towards the way we are now teaching and testing the clinical skills of the young people who will be our future physicians.... It is the thread that held the inspiration until all was ready for weaving – the golden winged rod entwined with oppositional energy that symbolizes the integration around which so much else has been explored and discovered. May that golden rod, now firmly planted, continue to inspire winged ideals ... to support the healers of today – and nurture those of tomorrow (Wallace, 1997, p. 18).

Adherence to a positivist perspective and empirical research questions has meant that no one has written about the OSCE in terms of its sociological functions; or its use in advancing the political or economic goals of the profession; nor indeed of any aspect of testing knowledge creation or power relations.

Foucault (1972-1977/1980) suggested that the most important aim of his research was to question those things that appeared to be "self-evident". Thus, it is seems reasonable to ask: Why should it be self-evident that the little OSCE that Harden invented in Scotland in 1975 would have or should have led to the examinations that process over 25,000 American medical graduates annually in five huge testing centres? Why should we think it inevitable that the classroom into which Paula Stillman first brought a lay person with a checklist to teach medical students would metamorphose into today's testing centres, where so much surveillance data is collected from video and audio recording that special air-conditioners are needed to deal with the heat from the dozens of computer servers? And why would we assume that the artist named Rose McWilliams, whom Howard Barrows first employed in the 1960s to pretend she had multiple sclerosis for his medical students, would be linked over time with the hundreds of professionalizing and unionizing standardized patients who grade the performance of students in multi-station examinations? Why would we imagine that these developments have one long and unbroken historical thread connecting them?

The challenge that I have taken in this research is to create a new history of OSCEs that could bring to light the conditions and contingencies that led to the birth and adoption of *various forms* and *uses* of OSCEs, without resorting to a linear, positivist narrative. The work of Michel Foucault provides a useful starting point for this research for two reasons: the first reason is epistemological and the second, methodological. At an epistemological level, Foucault was very interested in examinations. As I have noted, he viewed "the examination" as one of the most important tools invented in the classical age for the control of human behaviour. He saw a relationship between the behaviour-modifying effects of examinations in schools and the mechanisms of surveillance and control he studied in prisons and asylums. As he observed:

The examination combines the techniques of an observing hierarchy and those of a normalizing judgment. It is a normalizing gaze, a surveillance that makes it possible to qualify, to classify and to punish. It establishes over individuals a visibility though which one differentiates and judges them. That is why, in all the mechanisms of discipline, the examination is highly ritualized. In it are combined the ceremony of power and the form of the experiment, the deployment of force and the establishment of truth. At the heart of the procedures of discipline, it manifests the subjection of those who are perceived as objects and the objectification of those who are subjected (Foucault, 1975/1995, p. 184-85).

At a methodological level, Foucault's work is also very relevant. He wrote compelling genealogical histories of other technologies that construct knowledge and mediate power, such as the hospital, the classroom and the prison. Foucault argued that the history of such technologies (which he called "discursive objects") is rarely a unified trajectory of progressive refinement and development. Rather, he showed that such objects arise as a result of the existence of particular discourses that make them possible and that their nature and functions change as discourses change, assume dominance or disappear. This perspective, therefore, opens a door to research that explores the ways in which OSCEs have been, and are used for knowledge production and power at different times and in different places.

Although there are compelling Foucauldian analyses of the organization and governance of educational institutions in general (e.g. Popkewitz & Brennan, 1998), there are no existing publications that explore the OSCE, performance-based assessment, or simulated patients in this way. It is probably understandable that a post-structural analysis of this kind has not been attempted. As I have noted, positivist narratives of constant progress and objective reality are dominant in health professional education literature where new developments are framed as technological advancements based on scientific discovery and the march of progress.

In undertaking my research, I have employed the perspective that Foucault developed as a result of this own work; namely that history arises from a series of ruptures and discontinuities. My focus will be on the multiplicity of forms and uses of OSCEs. In exploring the extraordinary global reproduction of this technology, I hope to identify the major discourses that have made it possible, and the shifts and changes in those discourses that have led to its many variations. The value of this research at a theoretical level is to provide the first analysis of how a simple tool like the OSCE can become implicated in the creation of knowledge, in modifying the roles and positions available for individuals in medical education, and in the establishment and growth of institutions that mediate power.

1.4   My Location

I approach this research as an insider, having been involved in developing, studying, publishing about and, more recently, critically examining OSCEs. I experienced my first OSCE as a medical student, later took one for licensure and, as a junior faculty member, was involved in creating and running OSCEs for students at the University of Toronto. I have published articles on the use of the OSCE in my specialty of psychiatry and more generally for assessment of communication and inter-personal skills. I have served on test development committees for the Medical Council of Canada and the Royal College of Physicians and Surgeons of Canada. I continue to be involved in the use and study of OSCEs, although in recent years my research has shifted to become more critical, as I explore the limits and implications of their use. The research presented here, helped me to gain a deeper understanding of the social, economic, political, educational and ethical implications of using OSCEs. Re-examining OSCEs through a critical lens allows me to think and speak differently about the use of this simple but powerful technology. Muzzin has pointed out that, while a sizeable group of scholars in Canada are engaged in critical work examining universities and higher education in general, "little, or none of this activity has penetrated into our professional schools" (Muzzin, 2005, p. 152). I hope that my research will contribute something to this large gap in the research on professional assessment.

An important aspect of my research has involved reflecting on the ways in which my own history, contexts and relationships interacted with the data I gathered, and my interpretation of it. Sawicki (1991) made a strong case that the principal advantage of using a Foucauldian analysis is that one is forced to question all theoretical 'givens' as possibly being constrained by one's own embedded discourses. She argued that the researcher should reflect on his or her own discursive constraints and modeled how to do this by posing and responding to the following questions in her own work: Who are the "authors" of my discourse on Foucault and feminist theory? What conditions governed what could be said, how it could be said and whether I could say it? What were the political implications of the choices I made? What were the possibilities for resistance within the confines of my discipline? (Sawicki, 1991, p. 3)

Following Sawicki's model, I have tried to incorporate reflective analysis into my thesis. Donna Haraway's (1988) concept of "situated knowledges" is a reminder that particular "locations" (both physically and psychologically) make some ideas obvious and not others. I have tried to view the nature of these influences using the Foucauldian concept of subjectivity that I discuss in detail in Chapter 3. Briefly, Foucault felt that discourses make possible certain ways of thinking and of acting that he called "subject positions". In reflecting on my own history, I have tried to identify which subject positions I have taken up, and how these have made possible, or constrained my own perspectives. Foucault also felt that individuals create discourse; promoting and extending some statements, concept and strategies but not others. Thus, I have also tried to reflect on the way that I have been a "discoursing subject" and consider the nature of the discourses that I reproduce. Delhi has framed this as an effort to "think about the discourses and practices in which [one's] own research is constituted" (Dehli, 2003, p. 135).

This book is organized as follows: Chapter 2 is a review of the very limited work on examinations in medical education, followed by a review of socio-historical writing about examinations generally. Chapter 3 outlines the methodology of my research, describing the key elements of a Foucauldian socio-history. Chapter 4 begins the analysis with a detailed description of the search for "discontinuities" in OSCE history and the discovery and characterization of discursive formations. Chapters 5 to 7 are detailed explorations of three discourses -- performance, psychometrics and production -- including the statements, subject roles and institutions associated with each. Chapter 8 draws together the three discourses and explores their interrelationships as well as the implications at both individual and societal levels. Finally Chapter 9 concludes the thesis with reflections on what I hope will be the contributions of my research and its personal meaning and implications.

CHAPTER 2: THE EXAMINATIONS AND THEIR USES

2.0   Introduction

Three sets of literature were useful for framing this socio-historical study of OSCEs: histories of the OSCE; histories of the use of examinations in medical education (both "insider accounts" and sociological or historical studies); and works exploring examinations more generally. In this chapter, I review each of these literatures, summarize the main themes and examine the strength and weaknesses of previous works in terms of informing the design of a socio-history of the OSCE.

2.1   Histories of the OSCE

In Chapter 1, I cited a number of articles that provide details about the creation, modification, dissemination and evaluation of OSCEs. Taken together, this corpus of over 600 articles provides a history of sorts, although the vast majority of articles contain only a few lines about the individuals and institutions involved in the history of OSCEs. A few exceptions are the very frequent references to Ronald Harden who is credited in a number of articles with inventing the OSCE; to Howard Barrows who is frequently noted to have invented simulated patients; and to Paula Stillman whose name is, on many occasions, cited in relation to the invention of patient educators and behavioural checklists. Each of these individuals and their contributions are examined in the chapters that follow. A few articles provide some form of summary of the history of OSCEs. Nayer (1993), for example, wrote an article summarizing the invention, history and uptake of OSCEs for the purpose of introducing the technology to physiotherapists. Articles by van der Vleuten and Swanson (1990), Rothman and Cohen (1995) and Swanson and Stillman (1990) similarly take a somewhat broader perspective and provided an overview of the invention, adoption and adaptation of multi-station examinations and simulated patients. However, all of these articles have the flavour of technical writing and the goal of the authors, stated or implicit, was to help convey an understanding of how to use the technologies. The purpose of the articles is not to provide a history of the OSCE *per se*, and certainly not to write a critical one.

A few publications have a historical orientation. The first, a rather technical document, is a Masters thesis prepared at the University of Dundee for a degree in management. While the majority of the work was focused on the economic and business aspects of OSCEs, the author nonetheless provided a rudimentary analysis of how the OSCE arose and why, and how its use has been shifting in relation to educational and economic currents (Clark, 2000). The second, although largely a technical discussion of simulation and performance-based assessment, is the transcript of a speech given by George Miller (1990) in which he outlined the historical development and use of OSCEs and SPs. He also tied these inventions to a developmental model of learning -- the so-called "Miller's Pyramid", which subsequently became a widely used symbol for performance-based assessment. Third, the only attempt at a truly historical analysis of OSCEs and simulated patients is Peggy Wallace's (1997) publication *Following the Threads of Innovation: The History of Standardized Patients in Medical Education,* which recounted the history of simulated patients (and their renaming to standardized patients) as well as the history of OSCEs.

These three works provide a good overview of the individuals and locations involved in the appearance and uptake of OSCEs, as well as some of the important dates. Second, they provide some of the richest discourse for analysis. None of these authors, however, made any sociological observations about the history they presented, and all wrote in the upbeat, progressivist tone of positivism.

2.2   Histories of Examinations in Medicine

Beyond the OSCE literature, in the broader domain of medical education, there are two relevant literatures that contributed to my thinking about a socio-history of examinations. First there is a collection of books and papers that provide histories of medical examinations. These are mostly "insider" works written by physicians and medical educators, most often working for national educational or testing organizations. Second, there are general histories and sociological studies of medical education, written occasionally by physicians, but more often by historians and sociologists. I reviewed each of these with a focus on what they offered to a socio-historical study of OSCEs.

2.21 Insider Histories of the Use of Examinations in Medical Education

There is a collection of publications that document the development of certification examinations, particularly in North America. These yielded a number of important observations. For example, when medical schools moved into universities in the US, UK and Canada in the nineteenth century, examinations were initially the responsibility of each medical school, which issued a certificate of competence at the end of medical training (Shore & Scheiber, 1994). This remains the practice in some countries of the world such as France, where it is the name of the institutions from which students graduate that confers the qualification and prestige (Segouin & Berard, 2005). In North America and the UK, a system emerged that was more centralized and that would displace some of the power of individual medical schools. In the UK, this was the system of Royal Colleges that gradually emerged from various guilds and specialty organizations. During the twentieth century, these colleges elaborated the standards for training and conducted national examinations of competence that had to be passed in order to enter practice. In Canada, the Medical Council of Canada was founded in 1912 for certification of competence of graduates of Canadian medical schools (Dauphinee, 2004). At the post-graduate level, a single Royal College of Physicians and Surgeons of Canada (RCPSC) was founded in 1929 "to grant medical and surgical specialist certification by examination" (Burgess & Hurteau, 2004, p. 33). In the United States, there was nothing "royal"; however, the organizations that emerged were equally centralized and national in scope, and called "boards"; a terminology reflective of corporate governance. The American Board of Medical Specialties (ABMS) was founded to act as an umbrella for the various specialty boards which, like the Royal Colleges in the UK, set the national examinations for each specialty (Shore & Scheiber, 1994). The American Council on Graduate Medical Education (ACGME) was created to deal with national standards for residency training. Testing became the responsibility of special, independent testing organizations such as the Education Commission on Foreign Medical Graduates (ECFMG) and the National Board of Medical Examiners (NBME).

These organizations rose to prominence in the twentieth century, during which time the examination of future physicians came firmly under national, centralized control in all three countries. This had the effect of shifting discussions about what should be examined to a national level, leaving medical schools to implement curricula and in-training evaluation systems to support and prepare for the "high stakes" national examinations. As a result, almost all the histories of medical examinations are contained in books and articles written by "insider" authors who either worked for or consulted to these associations. Therefore, a link was often made between 'progress' in testing and institutional expansion. The Royal College of Physicians and Surgeons of Canada, for example, documented its history in a book entitled *The Evolution of Specialty Medicine,* in which a whole chapter was devoted to examinations (Dauphinee, 2004). The author noted that "the first steps in improving evaluation and examination for certification and licensure dealt less with measurement issues than with structures" and outlined how the development of the various testing organizations led to the reform of the process of examination. Dauphinee noted that the growth of testing organizations was linked to the emergence of "sufficient research capacity to ask questions about what we were doing". He cited the appointment of Arthur Rothman, an examination researcher at the University of Toronto in 1969, as the beginning of recognition that evaluation was "well suited to study and research" and of the collaboration between testing organizations and universities. In the 1970s and 1980s, a whole series of similar appointments of medical educators, researchers and psychometricians took place in medical schools across North America (Dauphinee, 2004, p. 114).

Similarly, Langley (1994) wrote a history of assessment by national organizations in the US, noting that specialty boards were developed "to define qualifications and issue credentials that would assure the public of the education and competence of the specialist". He cited one of the earliest calls for examinations by the American Academy of Ophthalmology and Otolaryngology, which argued in 1980 that one should not be licensed to practice without appearing before "a proper examining board" (Langley, 1994, p. 19). Similarly, in a book produced by the American Board of Psychiatry and Neurology entitled *Certification, Recertification and Lifetime Learning in Psychiatry,* Shore and Scheiber (1994) stated that the process of certification and recertification "achieved new momentum" in the 1980s as a result of "consumer demand, physician accountability, [and] economic factors that led to a change in patterns of practice", among others influences. Further, they insisted that "the public has renewed its demand for certification of physicians to ensure an acceptable standard of medical expertise" (Shore & Scheiber, 1994, p. 3). The definition of "the public" was "various third parties, insurance companies and government agencies" who were demanding certification and recertification. Shore and Scheiber noted that as of 1989, 23 American specialties boards had, or were developing processes of recertification (Shore & Scheiber, 1994, p.3). American sources documented the explosive growth in certification examinations in the 1970s and 1980s, noting that over 40 new certificates arose after 1980 alone, resulting in a total of over 70 American speciality and sub-specialty medical qualifications, each with its own examination (Langley, 1994).

Historical accounts by national testing organizations also touch on historical shifts in the nature of examinations that foreshadowed the OSCEs, as well as on the development of the institutions that run them. For example, Shore recounted the history of the shift from written examinations to performance examinations and documented the various "problems" with oral examinations (Shore & Scheiber, 1994). Similarly, the American Board of Medical Specialities (1981) produced a book entitled *Evaluation of Non-Cognitive Skills and Clinical Performance,* in which various medical specialities recounted the history of the development of assessment methods in their field, with a specific focus on the move away from the testing of knowledge towards performance-based assessment (Lloyd, 1982). To give but one example, Mankin provided an overview of assessment in orthopaedic surgery, highlighting the significant paradigm shift that occurred in the 1950s and 1960s when collaboration with Christine McGuire and George Miller at the University of Illinois in Chicago led to the first studies of performance-based assessment methods. Exposure to methods of simulation triggered "considerable soul searching" with regard to what constituted professional competence on the part of those involved, according to Mankin (1981, pp. 25-31).

Dauphinee underscored the centrality to the thinking of testing organizations of "Miller's Pyramid", a symbol he reproduced in his chapter (also reproduced in Chapter 5 of this thesis). The pyramid has at the bottom level the word "knows". At the next level appears the words "knows how", then "shows how" and finally, at the peak, the word "does". "Does" refers to the domain of what physicians actually do in practice. Declaring the need to test these performance aspects of competence opened

22

the door for assessment of fully trained physicians in practice. Examining the whole "sequence" of competence, according to Dauphinee, was "necessary for a valid evaluation process" (Dauphinee, 2004, pp. 112-113). Other histories written by testing organizations also place the development of assessment on a trajectory that aims for continuous testing of those in practice at the "peak of the pyramid". For example, as Shore and Scheiber (1994) noted, as early as 1940, a US Commission on Graduate Medical Education argued that it was desirable to issue to medical graduates time-limited certificates that would be renewed with further examinations. They documented how most US specialties went on to adopt the programs of continuous testing and recertification in use today.

To summarize this "insider" literature, the books and articles were all written in a similar style, using grand narratives that sweep the reader along an assumed trajectory of continual progress. They show how each event, discovery or invention led to ever more precise refinements of examination technology. Dauphinee, for example concluded that, "[t]he progress of evaluation within the medical profession in Canada over the last four decades is a good news story", he called it "a story of progress and innovation" (Dauphinee, 2004, p. 109). There are few critiques, although there were some subtle allusions to the idea that all the changes might not be 'progress'. One example is the history published by the American Board of Psychiatry and Neurology, the only board in the US to retain a 'live-patient' examination to the present day. While Shore and Scheiber (1994) recounted the standard history of the emergence of a science of psychometrics that rendered oral examinations 'unreliable', the articles in their book also subtly resisted the argument that validity should be primarily defined by psychometric reliability. In another example, Langley commented almost off-handedly in his history that "little evidence exists to prove that the certified specialist performs more effectively than the non-certified" (Langley, 1994, p. 28). Finally, none other than Christine McGuire, the author cited for her efforts to make examinations more psychometrically rigorous and who many credit with the discontinuation of oral examinations, wrote critically:

[S]ome sociologists maintain that further division of labour, increasing specialization and progressive bureaucratization of health care delivery will ultimately lead to a "deprofessionalization" or "de-skilling" of medical practice, reducing the role of the physician to that of technician, in a process not unlike that which gradually overtook craftsmen as a consequence of the industrial revolution (McGuire, 1994, p. 37).

But having worked this interesting quote from neo-Marxist Magali Larson into her chapter, McGuire made no further reference to these ideas and concluded by saying that "in the final analysis, relevant, objective, and valid data may be the only practical defence against what are certain to be growing professional, social and forensic challenges to certifying decisions" (McGuire, 1994, p. 47).

2.22   Perspectives on Examinations in Medical Education History and Sociology

In an article called entitled *The Many and Conflicting Histories of Medical Education* (2005), I published a review of histories of medical education written from many different perspectives including: positivist (Beck, 1850/1966, Norwood, 1970); political/economic (Starr, 1982); neo-Marxist (Brown, 1979; Johnson, 1972; Larkin; 1983; Larson, 1977;1980); critical feminist (Strong-Boag, 1981; Witz, 1992); and social-constructivist (Ludmerer, 1985; Bonner, 1995). This body of work was very helpful in illustrating shifts in the writing of medical history away from positivist/progressivist and towards critical/post-structural. It was also a useful guide to creating a more specific history of examinations, with many specific references to Canada as well as the United States and Europe. Unfortunately, among these histories of medical education, there are few specific references made to examinations since historians lumped examinations together with other technologies of medical education such as selection criteria and curricula. As I describe below, these historians were interested in the power of medical education, but few specifically explored the technology of examinations in that light. Nevertheless, it was useful to review this literature because it provides an excellent frame for some of the key elements of socio-history generally.

Not surprisingly, I found many conventional histories that document developments in medical education, such as the adoption in North American and the UK of the clinical methods of the Parisian clinical schools; the shift to clinical-pathological method; the rise of therapeutics, discipline-based research and clinical rotations; and the relocation of medical education to university settings (Beck, 1850/1966; Field, 1970; Flexner, 1925; O'Malley, 1970; Norwood, 1970). Examinations were sometimes mentioned as part of a brief description of the context or organization of medical school examinations. The only author to discuss examinations at some length was Abraham Flexner. His 1910 report was used to make dramatic changes to the structure of medical education in North America. While his report and the effects it had on medical education have been sharply critiqued (Brown, 1979), what he had to say about examinations appeared not to have had the same traction as his other recommendations. Said Flexner, "Examinations are necessary…but their importance, even as a protection to the public, may be over-emphasized; for the moment too much is made of them"; he argued that "too rigid examining therefore defeats its own end. In the long run, systems of education stand or fall by virtue of effort and ideas, not machinery" (Flexner, 1925, pp. 279-80). This comment foreshadowed the writings of the late twentieth century when large testing centres that worked very much like machines arose. While interesting as a historical footnote, Flexner's book did not provide any further analysis of examinations, and he, like the other conventional historians of medical education, left themes of professional power and examinations completely unexplored.

Authors with a neo-Marxist perspective, on the other hand, paid attention the uses of medical schools in terms of organization and financing; selection and recruitment of faculty; and selection of students in ways that served economic control of the profession and its social advancement. For example, in *Rockefeller Medical Men*, Brown framed the rise of the medical profession "from ignominy and frustrated ambition to prestige, power and considerable wealth" in economic terms and showed how the profession harnessed the momentum of capitalist society and rose to power by exploiting links to powerful philanthropic organizations such as the Rockefeller and Carnegie Foundations (Brown, 1979, p. 79). Similarly, Larson argued that medical education is a process that channels privilege and capital to a very select group of students. She wrote:
I see professionalization as the process by which producers of special services [seek] to constitute and control a market for their expertise. Because marketable expertise is a crucial element in the structure of modern inequality, professionalization appears

also as a collective assertion of special status and as a collective process of upward social mobility. (Larson, 1983, p. xvi)

Starr's (1985) *The Social Transformation of American Medicine: The rise of a sovereign profession and the making of a vast industry,* also provides an economic analysis of the way in which the medical profession rose from a small, non-influential trade to the most powerful of the professions. He saw the key role of medical education in that transformation, commenting that, "[t]he dream of reason did not take power into consideration….[T]he history of medicine has been written as an epic of progress, but it is also a tale of social and economic conflict over the emergence of new hierarchies of power and authority, new markets and new conditions of belief and experience" (Starr, 1985, p. 3-4). Authors with a political-economic perspective, including neo-Marxists, thus talked about power and knowledge creation. The instruments of power they analysed included acts of legislation, professional organizations, institutions and even medical curricula, but not examinations. Brown (1979) did mention the role of licensure in professional control, however, his focus was on licensure as a procedure and he gave scant mention to the technologies of examination on which licensure was based (Brown, 1979, p. 63-65).

Feminist historians such as Witz (1995) explored how male-dominated medical schools of the nineteenth and twentieth centuries used discriminatory admission polices, including examinations to.such an extent that women had to respond by opening their own schools. Similarly Strong-Boag's (1981) work, *Canadian Women Doctors: Feminism Constrained,* traces the history of the establishment and ultimate demise of these Canadian medical schools for women. She explored not only political issues, such as barriers to admission to medical schools, but also issues of curriculum. For example, according to Strong-Boag, women were offered much less science education at all levels, not just at university, in the belief that a science education would result in "de-sexed, feeble and arrogant female students…who would not take her 'proper place' in the social order" (Strong-Boag, 1981 p. 208).

Witz specifically explored the role of examinations in professional power. She discussed the use of examinations in "poaching" the jurisdiction of delivering babies from midwives by the medical profession. According to Witz, in 1800 a competent

26

physician gave purgatives and did blood letting, but certainly did not deliver babies. Yet only a few decades later, physicians in the UK and North America claimed that they were the only ones competent to perform deliveries. Witz wrote that the key means that physicians used to appropriate the competence of delivering babies from midwives was to incorporate the competence of obstetrics into medical licensure examinations. Witz's analysis thus points to the use of examinations as tools for political and economic ends.

A handful of other social-contextual histories explored how the history of medical education has been very different in various countries (Bonner, 1995; Ludmerer, 1985). Bonner, for example, wrote a comparison study of the history of medical education in the UK, France, Germany and the United States. Bonner's work included constructivist formulations of what medical education was and is in relation to specific contexts and noted that "familiar events in a single country looked different when viewed against a wider canvas" (Bonner, 1995, p. 5). The comparative lens allowed Bonner to make interesting observations that were absent from other histories and to explore the political and economic conditions that led to different historical developments in different countries. For example, Ludmerer (1985) explored medical education in North America and described a decline in the commitment of doctors to their social contract in relation to political and economic priorities of the profession. Despite the broad sociological approaches and the use of comparative/contextual lens in their analyses generally, however, neither Bonner nor Ludmerer extended their analysis to examinations.

Finally, there is a rich body of sociological work going back to the 1960s in which authors such as Eliot Friedson (1970) studied medical schools and their role in the socialization of medical students. Prominent writers in this area include Hafferty & McKinley (1993), Light (1993), Coburn (1993), Fox (1989) and Wolinksy (1993). While not historians, their contextually-based ethnographic research illustrates medical schools as subcultures that shape the medical profession. *Boys in White* (Becker, Greer, Hughes & Strauss, 1961) for example, provides a detailed portrayal of the atmosphere and exigencies of a teaching hospital in the 1960s and how these led to certain ways of thinking and behaving. Of all these works, only Becker et al. made mention of examinations. In *Boys in White*, he and his colleagues illustrated the effects of exams on medical students' behaviour. In addition to describing the nature of written and practice examinations observed during field work, they discussed issues such as the variability of examiner questioning, the ways in which tests could undermine learning, and the strategies students used to maximize their chances of passing (Becker et al., 1961, pp. 108, 275). *Boys in White* did not problematize examinations beyond this, however, and the authors noted that although "students are very frightened of them; they are, after all, an expected feature of school life" (Becker et al., p. 89). A few years later, Becker, Geer and Hughes (1968) published *Making the Grade*, an analysis of the effect of examinations in college generally. While this research clearly highlighted the degree to which students were driven by a desire to maximize their grade point average (GPA), the authors did not discuss the contingencies that held such a powerful examination culture in place.

More generally, Readings (1996) has written about how the adoption, by universities, of a corporate discourse of "excellence" can be linked to efforts to "raise standards". This line of inquiry could have opened the door to an analysis of examinations but this has not yet been done. Similarly, Gidney and Millar's (1994) history of professions at the University of Toronto and Muzzin's (2005) analysis of professional education and academic capitalism raise intriguing questions about how universities became so powerfully involved in controlling the access individuals have to professional training and practice. In these analyses, again, examinations appear as an implicit technology and not a specific object of study.

To summarize this literature, I found several passing references to, and observations of, examinations. But I discovered no historian or sociologist of medical education who took a specific interest in examinations.

2.23   Foucault and the Socio-History of Medical Examinations

There is, however, one compelling study of medical examination; Michel Foucault's *Birth of the Clinic* (1963/2003). In this work, Foucault traced the history of the emergence of clinical medicine and the examination of patients. He also suggested that similar contingencies led to the development of the clinical skills examination of students. According to Foucault, clinical teaching in medicine (as opposed to theoretical teaching) first appeared at Leyden in the Netherlands in 1658 and produced the first clinical professor, Boerhaave, whose students set up chairs and institutes of clinical medicine in Edinburgh in 1720 (Foucault, 1963/2003). This model was followed at universities in London, Oxford, Cambridge and Dublin. Foucault said, "In a very short time, this reform of the teaching system was to assume a much wider significance; it was recognized that it could reorganize the whole of medical knowledge.... A way of teaching and *saying* became a way of learning and *seeing*" (Foucault, 1963/2003, p. 77).

The shift to observation was accompanied by a change in both the practice of clinical medicine and also of how student competence was assessed. Testing the reproduction of knowledge was no longer sufficient without the performance of skills. Foucault noted that Pinel, for example, criticized unlimited questioning by examiners and strongly advised focusing on student medical history taking and physical examination. In Foucault's words, "[t]here is boundary, form, and meaning only if interrogation and examination are connected with each other, defining the level of fundamental structures the 'meeting place' of doctor and patient" (Foucault, 1963/2003, p. 136).

The development of formal clinical examinations of students may have first occurred in France. This is not surprising given that the oldest medical school was located there, established in 1220 at Montpellier. The clinical-pathological method (involving examination of patients) is also attributed to the French physician Laennec who invented the stethoscope (Shorter 1985). In *The Birth of the Clinic*, Foucault (1963/2003) traced the emergence of the examination of students in France. He noted that the decrees of Marly issued in March 1707 stipulated that medicine would be taught in all the universities of the kingdom, that students would receive their degree only after three years of study, and that "every year they would have to pass an examination before receiving the title of *bachelier*, *licencié*, or *docteur*" (Foucault, 1963/2003, p. 52).

Following the French Revolution, the medical profession was briefly dissolved but then quickly reconstituted by a revolutionary government that declared, "[y]ou will not re-establish guild-masterships, but you will require proof of capacity. One may become a doctor without having attended a school, but you will demand a solemn guarantee of the knowledge of every candidate" (Foucault, 1963/2003, p. 91). This was realized with legislation to "compel anyone who claims to practice one of the professions of the art of healing to undergo long studies and examination by a severe jury" (Foucault, 1963/2003, p. 93). The government required that "[t]he candidate doctor will expound at the patient's bedside the character of the species of disease and its treatment". Thus, "for the first time the criteria of theoretical knowledge and those of a practice that can be linked only to experience and custom were found together in a single institutional framework" (Foucault, 1963/2003, p. 93).

In another work, *Discipline and Punish*, Foucault (1975/1995) specifically discussed the technology of the examination and its role in disciplining individuals and society. Foucault himself never brought together his work on what he called, in *The Birth of the Clinic*, the "medical gaze" with his study of disciplinary examinations in *Discipline and Punish*. Indeed Hoskin (1993) has argued Foucault did not go far enough in emphasizing the centrality of examination technology in the transformation of education. Hoskin argued, "[w]here he [Foucault] saw a general shift in power-knowledge relations of which examination is a glittering part and where education is just one field among many, I now propose a specific shift in which examination lies at the heart of transformation" (Hoskin, 1993, p. 277). As I shall describe below, Hanson (1993) did take up this challenge in his comprehensive book *Testing Testing: The Social Consequence of the Examined Life*. I will review Hanson's work in detail, given its particular relevance to my research. However even Hanson did not tackle the topic of examinations in medical education.

2.3   Examinations as Technology

Casting the net more widely, I found several works that explored the history of examinations generally. The oldest reference I discovered was published in 1918 and was called *Examinations and Their Relation to Culture and Efficiency* (Hartog, 1918). Although published before critical history and sociology were popularized, Hartog nevertheless identified the power of examinations and wrote about their role in shaping the British Empire and its citizens. I make reference to his work below. Little else appeared on the topic in English until mid-century when Montgomery (1965) wrote *Examinations; An Account of Their Evolution as Administrative Devices in*

30

England. In this comprehensive overview of the use of examinations at all levels of British society, he wrote that "modern examinations" were "concerned with the very nature of society itself" (Montgomery, 1965, p. 242). He noted that although "the tremendous growth of examination systems in number size and influence is obvious to all... it is surprising that the broad evolution of large examination systems has not been considered" (Montgomery, 1965, p. ix). Until the 1980s, while manuals, guides and technical articles about examinations proliferated, virtually nothing was written from a socio-historical point of view. Rowntree (1987) wrote that:

it is easy to find writers concerned with how to produce a better multiple choice question, how to handle test results statistically, or how to compensate for the fact that different examiners respond differently to a given piece of student work. It is much less easy to find writers questioning the purpose of assessment, asking what qualities it does or should identify, examining its effects on the relationship between teachers and learners, or attempting to relate it to such concepts as truth, fairness, trust, humanity or social justice. Writers of the former preoccupation rarely give any indication of having considered questions of the latter kind. Insofar as they appear to regard assessment as non-problematic, their writing, though often extremely valuable in their way, gloss over more fundamental questions about whether what we are doing is the right thing and offer simply a technical prescription for doing it better (Rowntree, 1987, p. 2).

Sosnoski wrote a critique called *Examining Exams* in which he argued that "Foucault's analysis of discipline helps us to see the negative effects of exams are related to the way they punish and subjugate students" (Sosnoski, 1993, p. 306). However his paper is an analysis of examinations in literature. Finally, I discovered two very well researched, critical books on examinations. The first, Gould's (1981) *Mismeasure of Man* explored the rise of the use of quantitative measurements to classify individuals, beginning with a history of craniometry and others attempt to link measurable human characteristics to intelligence. Gould drew a line from these early 'scientific' studies to the twentieth century mass marketing of the idea of hereditary IQ and discussed its implications for social engineering and control. He also showed how developments in measurement led to a whole industry of standardized testing in North America. The second book was Hanson's (1993) *Testing Testing: The Social Consequences of the Examined Life.* This Foucauldian socio-history of examinations explored how examinations are used for control, discipline and the shaping of individuals in society. He created a genealogy of the "examined society" that linked many forms of assessment from drug screening, to nursery schools admission tests, to the civil service exams in China. These works are complemented by Rose's (1985) socio-history of the rise and legitimation of the discipline of psychology. In particular, the links Rose drew between the rising "scientific credibility, professional status and social importance" of the discipline and its development of tools of measurement to "diagnose, conceptualize and regulate pathologies of conduct" are helpful in framing the emergence of psychological measurement discourse in medical education (Rose, 1985, p. 226).

Hanson, Gould and Rose specifically tackled the uses of examinations as technology and who was using them for which purposes. The authors noted that the rise of examinations was linked to the aspirations of particular institutions or groups. Gould, for example, said that the rise of mass testing in the US (in particular, the IQ test and its variants) could be explained because the emerging profession of psychology wanted to demonstrate that "it could be as rigorous a science as physics"; that most "equated rigour and science with numbers and quantification"; and that "the most promising source of copious and objective numbers was in the embryonic field of mental testing" (Gould, 1981, p. 193). Further, he argued, "Psychology would come of age, and gain acceptance as a true science worthy of financial and institutional support, if it could bring the questions of human potential under the umbrella of science" (Gould, 1981, p. 193). Rose wrote that psychology "only began to establish itself as a functioning discourse when it abandoned the purity of anthropomorphic measures and dirtied its hands with the requirements of educational administration" (Rose, 1985, p. 230). Finally, Hanson drew links between the development of almost every screening and aptitude test in use in the United States and the military research undertaken to find a screening tool for recruits needed for the First World War (Hanson, 1993).

While Hartog, Montgomery, Hanson, Rose and Gould wrote at different periods of time and in different places, they described similar uses of examinations. I have grouped these into three themes: examinations to shape and control individuals; examinations to shape and control the nature of society; and examinations to serve

32

economic goals in neo-liberal society. These distinctions are not sharp and I do not mean to imply that an examination has only one of these uses. Indeed, all examinations probably have some role in each of these three functions depending on the conditions and context of their use.

2.31   Examinations to Shape and Control Individuals

The first examinations developed in the United Kingdom were juried examinations used by medieval craft guilds. The purpose of these examinations was for masters to judge the individual work of their apprentices (Hartog, 1918). When European medieval universities also started examining decades later, they did it in a manner analogous to the guilds (Hartog, 1918). The structure of university examinations consisted of panels of faculty members who conducted what would be recognized today as "oral examinations" to ensure the quality and depth of the learning of their students (Hanson, 1993). These examinations have been written about as designed to shape individuals and their knowledge, behaviour and attitudes in certain directions. Such examinations were not widely available; in fact access to them was highly restricted to members of a particular guild, profession or school.

In the UK, the first university written examination (in mathematics) took place at Trinity College Cambridge in 1702 (Morris, 1961). Both Cambridge and Oxford adopted examinations broadly after 1800 and during the nineteenth century, there was a veritable explosion of examinations in the UK. Kellett wrote in his 1936 autobiography, "if, in fact, I were asked what, in my opinion, what was an essential article of the Victorian faith, I should say it was 'I believe in Examinations'" (Roach, 1961, p. 3). Hartog wrote in the early twentieth century that "[e]very teacher, every administrative educational body knows that, whatever be the scheme and curricula, examinations do effectively control the class-rooms of our secondary schools and they control to a considerable extent our universities too" (Hartog, 1918, p. xiii).

Unlike the mass examinations described as shaping whole societies that I shall discuss below, British school examinations were created to guide individual students in different ways depending on their future vocational or professional role. Hartog commented: "The public demands that persons on whose service it relies, and for whose failures it cannot be compensated…should produce some certificate of competence based on an examination, and often on a series of examinations beginning in childhood and prolonged into early manhood and beyond" (Hartog, 1918, p. 2). A key element in the use of examinations to shape individuals was, he argued, repeated testing to continue to mould test takers in the desired direction. Thus, "teachers, lawyers, doctors, dentists, engineers, architects as well as civil, naval and military servants of the Crown" must be subject to their own continuous examinations with the effect that "their whole career is determined by such tests" (Hartog, 1918, p. 2).

In North America, the earliest record of an examination dates to 1646 at Harvard. Examinations were not common at that time in North America and were apparently strongly resisted by students during the colonial era (Hanson, 1993). Nevertheless, after 1800, as in Europe, examinations became widely used in universities across North America and entrance examinations were added in the late nineteenth century (Hanson, 1993). Examinations were also adopted in secondary and elementary schools. MacLeod (1982) wrote that competitive, written examinations came to exert "massive influence", constituting "possibly the single most intrusive and expensive innovation in Western education in the last century" (MacLeod, 1982, p. 16).

Hanson discussed at length the implications of this use of examinations for individuals. He insisted that "the contemporary concept of the individual is a product of the development and extension of examinations in the seventeenth and eighteenth centuries" (Hanson, 1993, p. 314). This formulation, which he credited to Foucault, did not mean that the concept of an individual did not exist prior to the seventeenth and eighteenth century, but rather that the constitution of individuals on the basis of physical, physiological and psychological dimensions was only possible as a result of a shift in which masses of data are collected on individuals and populations. This data, in turn was used to constitute what is normal, abnormal or deviant. Once such assessments were made possible and standards for normality are established, a whole set of diagnostic and therapeutic technologies and interventions were made possible (Hanson, 1993, p 314-316). Foucault's central focus in *Discipline and Punish* was to illustrate how these technologies of surveillance and normalization flourished in institutions such as hospitals, prisons and schools. Once these mechanisms were in place, he argued, the nature of individuals was not simply observed, tested or place under surveillance by the technology of examination, but *created* by it (Foucault, 1975/1995). Foucault's work, and Hanson's interpretation of it, make explicit the link between the use of examinations for surveillance and disciplining of individuals, and the larger project of shaping society as a whole. The next section will consider this use of examinations.

2.32   Examinations to Shape and Control the Nature of Society

Conditions favoured the emergence of examinations in Imperial China during the Chou Dynasty (1122-256 BC) and led to the creation of the first formal system of examinations during the Tang Dynasty (AD 618-907) (Elman, 2000; Hanson, 1993; Lai, 1970). The purpose of these examinations was to select nobles for the Imperial court. By about 1000 AD, China greatly expanded this system of "civil service examinations" and made the competition widely accessible. Amazingly, the form of examination developed under the Ming Dynasty (1368-1662) continued almost unchanged until the twentieth century (Franke, 1960). The Chinese Imperial examination system was central to the establishment of privilege in China for over a thousand years. Unlike Eurocentric countries which retained hereditary aristocracies well into last millennium, hereditary privilege virtually ceased in China by the time of the Sung Dynasty (AD 1000). In its place, a cadre of administrators and bureaucrats emerged to provide service to the Emperor in running the country. Although the selection of the Emperor himself followed hereditary lines, all other positions of power and prestige were determined by the results of these competitive examinations (Hanson, 1993).

The infrastructure required to implement such examinations was enormous, with as many as 20,000 people presenting for provincial examinations. Success at these qualified candidates to take further national examinations. In order to try to maintain examination security, examinations were held over three days and two nights in walled compounds within thousands of cubicles. No one could enter or leave and there was constant monitoring and security. Significant attention was given to examination security in the preparation and reproduction of examinations, searches of candidates, surveillance of writing and the marking of examination papers. There were elaborate attempts to try to circumvent examinations and many ingenious methods of cheating developed, including a whole industry designed to aid candidates, both in legitimate examination preparation and in cheating methods (Hanson, 1993, pp.188-190).

During the thousand years of this system of Chinese meritocracy (though always under the control of the emperor), it functioned to prevent the re-emergence of hereditary privilege (Elman, 2000; Hanson, 1993). Thus examinations were used as a technology to hold in place the social hierarchy of a large country. For over 500 years the traditional Chinese system "achieved harmoniously and smoothly, with almost no resort to force, a degree of intellectual homogeneity eagerly sought, but so far scarcely attained, by the most totalitarian systems" (Franke, cited in Hanson, 1993, p. 293).

According to scholars who studied the history of examinations in China such as Hanson, Lai, Franke and Elman, many conditions led to the discontinuation of the Chinese examination system in the twentieth century. Among these were discourses of Chinese nationalism and arguments that the demands of the tests (such as memorizing classical texts or writing poetry) were not particularly 'relevant' to the ability to govern the country (Hanson, 1993). Hanson pointed out that when change finally did occur, it was in concert with a series of international humiliations and foreign interventions in China that occurred during the early twentieth century. These, he said, led the Chinese government to 'modernize' in a way that would make the country more similar to Western foreign powers. Yet modernization apparently did not include a national system of examinations and thus the system was formally abolished by the empress dowager in 1905 (Hanson, 1993).

The Chinese examination was what would be called today a "selection examination". Selection examinations have many functions, but essentially operate as a gateway to opportunity and privilege. China was not the only country to use selection examinations to prevent the re-emergence of a hereditary aristocracy. Following the French Revolution, the Revolutionary government created the slogan "*A chacun selon son mérite*" (To each according to his merit). This idea still underpins the strong national systems of anonymous entrance testing for all professions in France (Kholer, Braun, Mari & Roland, 2003). As in China, the belief in France has been that the function of an examination system is to prevent the access to position by nobility or nepotism (Segouin & Hodges, 2006).

Hartog (1918) suggested that the Chinese civil service examinations also influenced the United Kingdom in the development of its own civil service examinations in the nineteenth century. Beginning around 1850 in colonies such as India and Egypt, the UK implemented examinations to rationalize the selection and appointment of civil servants. A theme running throughout the history of British civil service examinations in the nineteenth and twentieth centuries was their use to shape colonial citizens in ways consistent with the demands of the growing global empire. Hartog saw national examinations as a process that moulded what he called "the human material" that was "a matter of national and imperial concern" (Hartog, 1918, p. 3). While British civil service examinations were put in place to fend off "patronage" rather than inherited privilege (the later being alive and well in the UK during heyday of the Empire), a 1907 speech by the Earl of Cromer showed the degree to which examinations were considered important in preventing threats to the British Empire. According to Cromer, "the competitive system, whatever may be its defects, is greatly superior to that which is superseded". He warned darkly that "advocates of reform" must be cautious of changes that would revive "the abuses of the past" (Hartog, 1918, pg, 39). Similarly, in North America, examinations were used to form 'civilized' citizens and in particular to "acculturate an ever-enlarging immigrant population" (Sosnoski, 1993, p. 305).

In summary, there is a robust history of examinations being used for social engineering. Hanson described this use of examinations as the "realization of Saint-Simon's and Comte's utopian visions of the benefits to be realized by applying science to society" whereby testing could be used in order that "society would profit by making optimal use of its human resources" (Hanson, 1993, p. 210). So great has been the belief in the power of examination that societies as diverse as dynastic China, post-Revolutionary France and Imperial England have employed them to hold in place particular social regimes. Just as examinations have been considered a powerful technology to shape and discipline individuals, so examination systems on a mass scale have been considered powerful technologies for shaping and disciplining societies. Now I will turn to what these authors wrote about the purposes this panoply of examinations was created to serve in twentieth century North America.

2.33   Examinations as Tools to Serve Economic Goals in Neo-Liberal Societies

A growing body of literature in professional education addresses the rise of academic capitalism in higher educational institutions in the twentieth century (Magnusson, 2000; Muzzin, 2005). For example, Dhruvarajan (2005) has highlighted the explicit role of universities in the dispersion of neo-liberal, capitalist ideas. She wrote, "in North America, students are carefully trained in the tenets of this paradigm". This, according to her, is a result of the discourse which positions globalization as the "only way" and that a "new world order has to be ushered in". In that new world, "to be free is to have free trade and to have democracy means unfettered conduct for corporations" (Dhruvarajan, 2005, pp. 135-137). Both books on examinations that I reviewed provide evidence that examinations are part of neo-liberal industrialization and globalization.

Examination became the target of a massive research and development process in the twentieth century in the United States. Both Hanson (1993) and Gould (1981) argued that the goal of this research was to make examinations more scientific, but also to render them more efficient tools for political and economic purposes. A vivid example was the project that fused the interests of the emerging profession of testing psychologists, who use large bodies of standardized, quantitative data to study intelligence, with pre-World War I American military goals. An ideal opportunity presented itself in the realm of examination research and served both groups well. The military wanted a test to screen millions of recruits for the First World War. The problem was that the only available format for testing intelligence was the cumbersome Binet test invented in France to assess developmentally delayed children. Further, the Binet test had been developed for the purpose of adapting education for students with learning difficulties and was administered individually to children by trained technicians (Gould, 1981, p. 152). Two research projects allowed the French test for learning-disabled children to be adapted for the screening of millions of military recruits in the United States. First, Lewis Terman, a professor at Stanford University who "dreamed of a rational society that would allocate

38

professions by IQ scores", adapted the test for adults and called it the Stanford-Binet Intelligence Test (Gould, 1981, p. 157). Second, the cumbersome and time consuming individually administered test was replaced with multiple-choices questions, invented in 1915 by Frederick J. Kelly (Hanson, 1993). The fusion of the multiple-choice format and the adult version of the IQ test led to the creation by Yerkes of the "Army Alpha", a test that was administered to 1.75 million men in the US army in World War I. Gould noted that the "supposedly objective data" amassed as a result of the army alpha work was then used to support restrictive immigration policies by embedding conceptions of racial and cultural inferiority in the Immigration Restriction Act of 1924 (Gould, 1981, p. 157).

Research on examinations was not, however, confined to one military project. At universities in America there has been, since the nineteenth century, "a widespread desire to bring some consistency to college entrance procedures" (Hanson, 1993, p. 214). This led first to the formation of a common College Entrance Examination Board (CEEB), which in 1900 replaced an array of smaller entrance examinations administered by individual universities. In the US, power was transferred to the CEEB when universities agreed to recognize its examination results in making their admissions decisions (Hanson, 1993). With the success of the Army Alpha, the CEEB saw the opportunity for an even more efficient testing of aptitude; thus the Army Alpha was once again modified and a new test called the Scholastic Aptitude Test (SAT) was born (Gould, 1981; Hanson, 1993).

While the SAT was pronounced to be "free from discrimination" for students who attended "inferior high schools", its widespread adoption led to the discovery of significant cultural, racial and gender biases (Hanson, 1993). For example, its core scientific assumptions were shown to confound inherent traits with culture, socio-economic level and environment (Gould, 1981). These observations were consistent with the work of sociologists who theorized IQ testing as a process of distributing privilege. Basil Bernstein (1990), for example, wrote that many pedagogical technologies, including examinations, serve to produce cultural and class disparities. In his work, *Class, Codes and Control: The Structuring of Pedagogic Discourse,* he wrote: "New forms of assessment [and] profiling" are "allegedly [created] to recognize and liberate individual qualities" but are, in fact, "new distribution procedures for homogenizing" (Bernstein, 1990, p. 10).

The use of examinations as political-economic tools was institutionalized in the US in 1947 when a new organization, called the Education and Testing Service (ETS), was established as a (non-profit) corporation. Through a series of acquisitions and corporate growth, it took over most of the work of designing and administering tests from the CEEB and further universalized and standardized the use of the SAT in almost all educational settings in the US (Gould, 1981). Today almost every mass test of selection or psychological testing and many tests of performance used in the United States can trace its roots to the SAT, a mass testing technology that is owned and operated by a corporation (Hanson, 1993).

During the twentieth century then, testing greatly accelerated. However, as illustrated in Rowntree's (1987) observation, there was a tremendous proliferation of writing about the technical aspects of assessment in the absence of any sociological critique. Meanwhile, by the mid-twentieth century, the examination was becoming a highly refined "administrative technology" (Rose 1985) that was as important to governmentality of neo-liberal, capitalist society as the factory or the prison.

2.4   Summary

A broad review of the socio-historical literature on examinations provided much more context than the simple histories of the OSCE published by medical insiders in medical education journals. What was hidden from view in the insider articles was the degree to which ways of thinking about and constructing OSCEs were imported from other discursive fields. Authors such as Gould, Hanson and Foucault provided a context for understanding examinations as technology -- technology that can be put in the service of quite different goals depending on the society in which it is employed. In late twentieth century neo-liberal America, Canada and the UK, examinations were tools linked to economic and political priorities such and the 'rationalization' and privatization of education; the restriction of access to certain groups; the erosion of the welfare system as it related to education; a concomitant surge in fees for tuition

40

but also for examinations; and with the emergence of new imperatives of measurement, accountability and research linked to the goal of generation of capital.

With this overview in mind, I set out to explore the more specific history of multi-station, performance-based OSCEs. My approach has been to explore these histories in whatever specificity might be reasonable, trying never to lose sight of the larger context in which they emerged. In keeping one eye trained on this larger context, so to speak, I hope I have avoided the error of invoking the autochthonous emergence of the OSCEs as though it were a comet appearing from a completely black night.

CHAPTER 3: FOUCAULDIAN METHODOLOGY

3.0   Introduction

I shall accept the groupings that history suggests only to subject them at once to interrogation; to break them up and then to see whether they can be legitimately reformed; or whether other groupings should be made; to replace them in a more general space which, while dissipating their apparent familiarity, makes it possible to construct theories of them (Foucault, 1969/1972, p. 26).

This chapter describes the methodology of my research. First I outline the nature of Foucauldian historical research and the key concepts of archaeology, genealogy and serial history. Next I describe the sources of data ("the archive") and decisions I made about the parameters of data collection. Finally, ethical issues in the research are discussed.

3.1   Overview of Foucauldian Method: Archaeology, Genealogy, and Discourse

3.11   Serial History and Total History

This research is historical and thus concerned with discovering and documenting "stories" of the Objective Structured Clinical Examination. As noted, I have approached my research using a framework inspired by the work of Michel Foucault. In particular, I have based my work on his conception of the nature of discourse elaborated in *The Archaeology of Knowledge* (Foucault, 1969/1972) and in a series of socio-histories (*Madness and Civilization,* 1961; *Birth of the Clinic,* 1963; *History of Sexuality, Volumes 1-3,* 1976/1990, 1984/1990 & 1984/1988; and *Discipline and Punish* 1975/1995). To use such a framework is to try to articulate what Foucault called a "serial history", rather than a traditional "total history" (Foucault, 1967/1998). He described the latter as a continuous, linear and generally progressivist story, and noted that it is the usual way of recounting history. A serial history, on the other hand, is one of layers, series and disruptions linked to different discourses that struggle for dominance at different times and in different places. Foucault wrote:

In traditional history it was thought that events were what was known, what was visible, what was directly or indirectly identifiable, and the work of the historian was to search for their cause or their meaning.... Serial history makes it possible to bring out different layers of events as it were, some being visible, even immediately knowable by the contemporaries, and then, beneath these events that form the froth of history, so to speak, there are other events that are invisible, imperceptible for the contemporaries, and are of completely different form (Foucault, 1972/1998, pp. 427-428).

Attention to disruptions rather than continuities and to series and layers rather than to a unified narrative means that a serial history is more an elaboration of the jostling of competing discourses and their links to various "regimes of truth" than is it a single, progressivist story of invention and refinement. Not only are shifts and ruptures accorded a place in a Foucauldian history, they are accorded primacy.

In order to further clarify the nature of Foucauldian genealogical history, it is useful to examine examples from Foucault's own work. Foucault undertook genealogical studies in order to create new socio-historical interpretations of specific discursive phenomena. Such phenomena were usually previously described in accounts that were accepted or 'understood' as a result of the singular telling of their histories. In creating a genealogy that would retell a familiar story in a new way, Foucault first sought out the appearance of a phenomenon, or what he called a discursive object. Some examples he studied were 'madness', 'criminality' and 'sexuality'. He carefully studied the nature of each discursive object, elaborating in great detail the twists, turns and interconnections of its nature and evolution. His goal was to show how a particular set of "statements" brought the discursive object into existence in a particular way. Using this approach, he produced fresh and surprising genealogies of sexuality, madness and criminality, among others.

Because a genealogy is a serial rather than a total history, a Foucauldian genealogist does not accept previously defined historical periods but rather strives to elucidate the origins and development, but also the ruptures and discontinuities in a story that may at first appear to be continuous. Thus, in tackling 'madness', Foucault was careful not to write a history of 'mental illness' or of 'psychiatry' -- two specific discourses that already contained within them circumscribed and limiting theoretical understandings of madness (Foucault, 1961/1988). Rather, he sought the origins of madness as an object, and tried to chart the various conceptualizations of it (evil or spiritual occupation, deviation form a behavioural norm, sickness or illness, etc.) during different periods of history. In this way he showed that psychiatry and its concept of 'madness-as-illness' is simply one formulation of madness that appeared during a specific period of time. The twentieth century discourse of 'madness-as-illness' could not be understood without the intersecting discourses of psychiatry, medicine, medication, treatment, fitness to work in the labour force, etc.

Similarly, in Volume 1 of *The History of Sexuality,* Foucault (1976/1990) showed that the common conception of the Victorian Era as sexually repressive is an inverted formulation and that, in fact, the mechanisms of 'repression' during the Victoria era actually produced quite the opposite effect. According to his analysis, during the Victorian era, a plethora of sex laws, trials and prohibitions actually expanded the discourse of sexuality to a level of fervour not previously seen in British history.

Addressing criminology in his book, *Discipline and Punish,* Foucault (1975/1995) showed how the 'humanitarian reforms' of prisons in the nineteenth and twentieth century were actually a shift from an externalized system of punishment and torture, to an internalized system of self-control and self-directed punishment, whereby every citizen is monitored by an architecture -- both material and psychological -- that controls his or her behaviours and thoughts.

Turning to a twentieth century discursive formation, the Objective Structured Clinical Examination, my research explores the relationship of its appearance and legitimation with other discursive objects and concepts such as 'performance-based assessment', 'psychometric reliability and validity', 'standardization' and 'production', among others. I have not uncritically accepted the oft-repeated statements that the OSCE was the 'inevitable' product of a demand for reliable assessment, or the 'need' to address doctor-patient relationships, or an 'imperative' to safeguard the public from incompetent doctors. In the words of Kendall and Wickham, "[w]hen we describe an historical event as contingent, what we mean is that the emergence of that event was not necessary, but was one possible result of a whole series of complex relations between other events" (Kendall & Wickham, 2003, p.5).

To speak about the Objective Structured Clinical Examination in these terms, then, would be to show that it arose at a particular period of time, in a particular location in relation to a number of contingent discourses. The OSCE can be seen as arising as certain discourses created favourable conditions for its emergence. However, I am working from the assumption that the phenomenon of OSCEs is not a continuous construct. Instead, I assume that at different times and in different places, what an OSCE *is*, relates to the underlying discourse(s) that make it possible, propel its use and dissemination and give it a particular character. It is not sufficient simply to write a story of an increasingly sophisticated innovation, refined by more understanding, more research and more development. On the contrary, it is assumed here that what the OSCE *is* constantly shifts, changes and metamorphoses as its foundational discourses shift and metamorphose.

As I have suggested in the previous chapter, the OSCE itself is only a tool. However, I will argue that it is a tool harnessed to important discourses related to knowledge production, which, in turn relate to power. The OSCE itself has been passed across the discontinuities of various emerging, dominant or receding discourses and survives each time only in so much as it can be made to serve the knowledge production/power needs of the dominant discourses to which is it harnessed. Because there are multiple competing discourses at any given time, I will argue that there are struggles to define and to control what an OSCE is and how it is used. Discontinuities are signalled by efforts that find new uses for it, to discredit other uses of it or to shift its use into new areas. Such disruptions may be seen to trigger resistance, particularly when a new discourse is emerging or assuming dominance.

The historical beginnings and ends of discourses are not finite and their chronological limits cannot be fixed precisely. Neither can they be said to be linear in their appearance and disappearance. Further, when a particular discourse rises to prominence and another can be seen to fade, there is no certainty that they do so in lock step. Thus several discourses can exist simultaneously. Nevertheless, broad periods can be defined during which discourses appear, rise to dominance, and pass into unquestioned "regimes of truth" that are later displaced by new and emerging or re-emerging discourses. These transitions are marked by discontinuities, and it is these discontinuities that are the focus of a Foucauldian genealogy. Discontinuities

45

are rarely neatly tied to major historical dates, or events, but rather may be heralded by a shift in language or behaviour, by the appearance of an article or idea, or simply by a moment when a once-resisted argument passes for the truth. I will argue that the history of the OSCE is characterized by several of these discontinuities and it is the focus of my research to elucidate them in order to identify the key discourses that have arisen, predominated and declined. Thus Foucault's method and mine is "a problem-based rather than a period-based approach" (Kendall & Wickham, 2003, pg. 23). Foucault wished to begin with no single, unitary pre-existing organization -- no force, tradition, argument or theory whose existence must be taken as *the* antecedent and therefore as *the* constituting factor for the discursive formations under study.

3.12   Conducting a Foucauldian Discourse Analysis

The methodology I have used to approach the data is anchored in an approach broadly called critical discourse analysis. Critical discourse analysis has roots in the work of a number of philosophers of language and social theory such as Bakhtin (1981), Pecheux (1975) and Wittgenstein (1953), as well as Foucault (1969/1972), who assumed that language is socially constructed and helped break with the structuralist traditions of linguistic analysis. Critical discourse analysis grew out of this work and developed important momentum as a research approach after the 1970s as part of the so-called "linguistic turn" in the social sciences. Three intellectual traditions -- discourse studies, feminist post-structuralism and critical linguistics -- were particularly important in focusing on the relation of language to the construction of social phenomena and extended the use of discourse analysis into many fields of inquiry, including education (Rogers, Malancharuvil-Berkes, Mosley, Hui & O'Garro, 2005). What unites all methods of critical discourse analysis, and distinguishes them from other models of discourse analysis, such as traditional linguistic analysis, is their "movement from description and interpretation to explanation of how discourse systematically constructs versions of the social world" (Rogers et al., 2005, p. 371).

Thus, while there are different approaches to critical discourse analysis, all involve exploring the relationship between two levels of language: actual texts (usually involving a close reading of textual materials, including those derived from speech) and analysis of the macro-sociological *use/context* of that language. All methods of

46

critical discourse analysis have developed some means of moving between textual/linguistic analysis and larger social discourse. Foucault's work is classified with the French discourse method (Rogers et al., 2005). In characterizing this approach of discourse analysis, it is helpful to contrast it with other related but different approaches.

The method developed by Norman Fairclough is the most commonly reported method in critical discourse analysis research in education in North America (Rogers et al., 2005). Fairclough articulated this method in his book *Language and Power* (1989) and further refined his methodological approach in two subsequent books (Fairclough, 1995; 2003). Briefly, Fairclough's analytic framework is constituted by three levels of analysis: the text, the discursive practice, and the sociocultural practice. In other words, each discursive event has three dimensions: It is a spoken or written text, it is an instance of discourse practice involving the production and interpretation of texts, and it is a part of social practice. The analysis of text involves the study of the language structures produced in a discursive event. An analysis of the discursive practice involves examining the production, consumption and reproduction of the texts. The analysis of sociocultural practice includes an exploration of what is happening in a particular sociocultural framework (Rogers et al., 2005, p. 371).

It is important to note that this method *begins* with textual material and moves *towards* an ever-widening field where language is used in social contexts. Fairclough understands this as an extension of linguistic analysis beyond its previous structuralist method that would have stopped at the textual analysis stage.

By contrast, while Foucault was also very interested in texts, his method is not a unidirectional analysis from text to discursive practices to social practices. Fairclough himself noted that, although his approach is very compatible with that of Foucault, his is 'textually oriented discourse analysis' (TODA). For Foucault, however, the distinction between speech (parole) and language (langue) was not sufficiently explanatory to allow an analysis at one level to be extrapolated to another (Rogers et al., 2005). He did not feel that discursive formations arose solely from text, and described the difference between what he called "statements" and the more structural

47

concepts of sentences and propositions given by grammar and logic respectively (Foucault, 1969/1972).

Rather, Foucault's focus was to explore, critique and dismantle constructs that might be considered 'natural' (madness, justice, normality, sexuality, etc.) and show how such constructs are the product of power/knowledge relationships which are not only founded on a series of repeated and legitimized statements, but reciprocally make those statements possible (Rogers et al., 2005). Thus, Foucault focused on all the levels of discourse (he described four: discursive objects, statements/enunciative modalities, concepts and strategic choices -- discussed in detail later) that bring into existence the construct of interest. The textual level is important, but it is neither the starting place, nor a level of discourse that can be abandoned once the researcher moves to the higher social level. Foucault felt that social practices and their links to power/knowledge constrain the production and use of text (as well as speech). While speech and text construct discourse, discourse makes certain forms of text and speech possible (and others less possible). Thus, the two must be studied in an iterative fashion. In the research presented here, I have used the Foucauldian idea of an interactive approach to defining discourse, moving between the social and the text, rather than Fairclough's uni-directional approach.

Foucault developed two terms for the process of analysis at the micro-textual level (although he never remained at the level of grammar/linguistic structure alone) and for the macro-sociological level. The first, he called archaeology. Interestingly, he allowed for a certain degree of structuralism in an archaeological analysis. His archaeology has been called a "strict analysis of discourse" that tries to take a neutral position and avoid causal theories of change (Dreyfus & Rabinow, 1982, pp. 104-5). Genealogy, on the other hand, tries to locate and characterize the constituting power of discourse. It includes attention to dissenting opinions and theories (those that do not become widely recognized or established) as well as local beliefs and knowledge. A genealogy attempts to bring these opinions, arguments and knowledge into view. Foucault said, "Let us give the term genealogy to the union of erudite knowledge and local memories which allow us to establish a historical knowledge of struggles and to make use of this knowledge tactically today" (Foucault, 1972-1977/1994, p. 42). Whereas an archaeology is a study of the practice of language, genealogy uncovers

48

the creation of objects through institutional practices (Dreyfus & Rabinow, 1982, p. 104). A purely archaeological historian might claim to write from a neutral or 'disinterested' position, whereas a genealogist writing in the Foucauldian tradition will be aware of, and admit to political or polemical interests that motivate the writing of history (Hoy, 1986, pp. 6-7). In practice, if one is using a Foucauldian method it is probably not possible to create 'pure' archaeologies given that the aim is to move back and forth in an iterative fashion between the level of linguistic analysis and the level of social analysis. Thus Foucault's works generally have both archaeological and genealogical elements. My research contains the terminology and methods of both archaeology (the more structural analysis presented in chapter 4, for example) and genealogy (beginning with issues of knowledge creation and power in chapters 5 to 7). Overall the detailed analysis of the play of power at both individual and institutions levels that permeate this research make it most like the genealogies that I have described earlier.

3.2   Data Collection

Rogers et al. (2005) criticized much critical discourse analysis research in education for its scanty articulation of the analytic method used. They argued that it is well and good for a researcher to resist methods that reproduce positivist and structuralist methods rejected after the linguistic turn. But they argued that it remains important for the researcher to explain how the analysis preceded, what assumptions and methods were used, and to be reflexive about the role of the researcher him or herself in selecting the approaches.

Foucault noted that, as a result of the apparent unity of history and the pull to tell "totalizing" versions of it, the genealogist "is confronted by a number of methodological problems" (Foucault, 1969/1972, p. 10). He suggested the importance of:

1. identification and documentation of the sources of information to be used (which he called building up a coherent "corpora" of documents)
2. delimitation of groups and sub-groups that articulate the material (including specifying regions and periods of study)
3. establishment of principles of choice as to how these should be examined

4. specification of a method of analysis (such as breaking down the material according to a number of assignable features whose correlations are studied) (Foucault, 1969/1972, p. 10)

I have used these four principles to structure my research. What follows is an outline of some of my central methodological decisions, findings and analysis.

3.21 Identification, Documentation and Delimitation of Sources of Information

Foucauldian research involves investigating an "archive" that is the representation of the set of discourses of interest (Foucault, 1969/1972, p. 290). Because a discursive archive is coextensive with, but much more than just textual documents, I sought to capture and analyze discourse from three sources: the literature (textual), interviews with key informants (verbal/textual), and institutional data (verbal, textual and observational). I conceptualize these three sources -- literature, key informants and institutions -- as "sites" where the discursive elements could be located and characterized including "objects", "discoursing subjects" and "surfaces of emergence" through which discourses are expressed, reproduced and reinforced.

An immediate challenge was to delimit the sources of information in such a way that they were manageable, yet not restrict them so much that they might be reduced to an impoverished archive that might limit the identification of discursive formations. Prior to beginning my research, I set parameters and throughout the research I made minor modification in order that I might enlarge the field of study when necessary to better understand historical details or a discursive element. These modifications are summarized in Table 1 below.

Table 1: Delimitation of Sources of Information

	Initial decision	Modifications
Sources	Literature, interviews and institutional visits	Two additional sources of data added: • Presentations given at international conferences (documented in abstracts as well as field notes) • Autoethnographic elements (the idea that discourse is "inscribed" in my own history)
Dates	1975 (Harden's invention of the OSCE) to present	Review of examinations went back to 200 BCE. Expanded the OSCE history to include the 10 years from 1964-1974 that included the invention of simulated patients and their variations.
Language	English language	Addition of French sources.
Locations	Anglo-Saxon medical schools and testing organizations	Restricted to five main sites: UK (Dundee), Canada (Toronto, Montreal and Hamilton) US (Philadelphia). I also examined the extensive materials related to the uptake of OSCEs around the world.

3.3 Principles and Methods of Analysis

3.31 Literature

The question posed by language analysis of some discursive fact or other is always: according to what rules has a particular statement been made, and consequently according to what rules could other similar statements be made? The description of the events of discourse poses a quite different question: how is it that one particular statement appeared rather than another? (Foucault, 1969/1972, p. 27).

As I have discussed in detail above, Foucault used text extensively in his own research, but critiqued the traditional historical approach to text as inadequate for genealogical discourse analysis. He felt that this traditional approach was overly preoccupied with questions about "whether they were telling the truth" and "whether they were sincere or deliberately misleading, well informed or ignorant, authentic or tampered with" (Foucault, 1969/1972, p. 6). He suggested that the primary task of the historian was instead to "define within the documentary material itself unities, totalities, series, relations" (Foucault, 1969/1972, p. 6). In other words, he argued that one should not question the *accuracy* of texts but rather should examine a given text as an example of a set of statements, which are made possible by certain discourses. Foucault believed that "discoursing subjects", such as the authors of texts, are able to make some statements but not others according to rules that govern what is possible and legitimate to express. These rules of formation are the sign posts to the existence of specific contingent discourses.

To begin, Foucault recommended a "pure description of discursive events as the horizon for the search for the unities that form within it" (Foucault, 1969/1972, p. 27). By this he meant not an analysis of language (as I discussed above) but rather an attempt to answer the question "how is it that one particular statement appeared rather than another?" (Foucault, 1969/1972, p. 27). The search for repeated key words and metaphors, for recurring arguments and for shifts in the nature of those arguments (for example from a statement of opinion or possibility to a statement of fact) provides a rich data set from which to begin to define discursive systems.

52

The first source of data I studied was the published literature related to OSCEs and health professional education. This analysis was based on the University of Dundee compilation of close to 900 articles published in English between 1978 and 2005. In order to analyze such an extensive literature in an effective and efficient manner, I employed a focused technique. Two types of information were sought. First, the papers were arranged to create a historico-geographic mapping of where and when OSCEs appeared in the last 30 years. The second technique involved a focused content analysis. Each paper was analyzed for key words, embedded metaphors, key arguments and thresholds and shown in Table 2 below.

Table 2: Coding Guide for Literature

Location, date, funding

Location: Where do arguments come from? What institutions, professions, countries?

Date: Is there a shift over time in the people or institutions writing or speaking about OSCEs?

Funding: Who invests in OSCEs? What else do they fund? Where do they get their money?

Social elements

Who is authorized to write and speak about OSCEs? What education/degrees do they have? Does writing advance their careers? Do they know each other? How do they share ideas and interact?

Key words and metaphors

What key words recur in papers and transcripts? Is there a change over time? Do certain words or ideas disappear over time? What metaphors are used to talk about OSCEs? What societal discourses do these reflect?

Key arguments and thresholds

What arguments are used for adoption (or rejection) of OSCEs? To what philosophies, perspectives or agendas are they linked? Do they change over time? When do 'arguments' become 'truths'?

Data collection began with the database of articles referenced in the Dundee OSCE registry. As many of these articles as possible were retrieved and additional articles identified from secondary sources were added. I randomly pulled articles in groups of 10 and reviewed them using a coding face sheet to facilitate identification and collection of key discursive elements in each paper. During this process I created a historical timeline with key events, visits, conferences, and so on noted. This set of historical events is shown in Appendix A. I was particularly interested in identifying discontinuities, a phenomenon I have discussed at length in Chapter 4. Not all papers were reviewed in depth. On examining the title and abstract, if the information was already well covered in other articles, only the author, location and other demographic information was noted for the historical mapping. Detailed results of the literature analysis will be presented in chapter 4.

3.32   Interviews

Foucault is credited (or critiqued) for "decentring the subject". He did not deny the existence of individual subjectivity, but argued that discourses make possible a limited number of "subject positions" and that individuals who occupy these positions contribute to the perpetuation of discourses that made their subjective positions possible. [2] He explained that "the positions of the subject are also defined by the situation that it is possible for him to occupy" (Foucault, 1969/1972, p. 52). While not denying the possibility of agency, he did feel that thought and actions are constrained by possibilities created, or made difficult by, certain discourses. At the same time, I wanted to examine what Smith called the "local practices of the discourse" that allow the researcher to, in her words, "lift the discourse off the page and pull it into life" (Smith, 2004, p. 134). In chapters 5 to 7, I will discuss various forms of resistance that can be identified as responses to the dominant discourses I have identified. It is through these resistances that individuals engage agency.

As I noted above, in order to describe the nature of subjective positions that arose or disappeared in relation to various OSCE discourses, I undertook a series of individual interviews. Participants were first selected for their visible role in the history of OSCEs (for example, as authors of papers, conference speakers, directors of OSCE test centers, and so on). Later I added participants who would help me understand and

---

[2] Here I use the word "subject position" as did Foucault to mean a way of thinking, acting and being as a result of a discourse. I do not use the word "subject" as it is used in the experimental tradition to name individuals from whom data is collected. These individuals, who were active in helping me understand the discourses that affected them, I have called "participants" or "informants" in my research.

interpret the nature of discursive statements that emerged during the literature analysis.

Foucault described the essential questions in approaching "discoursing subjects":

"Who is speaking? Who, among the totality of speaking individuals, is accorded the right to use this sort of language? Who is qualified to do so? Who derives from it his own special quality, his prestige, and from whom, in return, does he receive, if not the assurance, at least the presumption that what he says is true?" (Foucault, 1969/1972, p. 50)

Based on this, I used my interviews for two major purposes. The first was to collect from a non-literature source, examples of discursive statements to add to those extracted from the collection of OSCE articles. There were some important differences between interviews and published texts that allowed me to confirm, extend, modify or reject some of the conclusions I was drawing from the literature. For example, there were constraints on interviews such as expectations about the relationship between the interviewer and interviewees, the social desirability of responding in certain ways, and the technical aspects of capturing non-verbal expressions. Despite these constraints, it is important to acknowledge that published texts are even more filtered through extensive and potentially distorting reviewers and editors who alter the nature of what is said. Second, live interviews allowed ideas and formulations to be introduced and reacted to by participants in a way that historical documents did not allow. An example is how difficult it would have been to guess the opinion of OSCE inventor Ronald Harden about the replication of the OSCE around the world by reading his papers alone; in my interview with him, I simply asked. Finally, the iterative nature of interviewing allowed for the presentation of hypotheses for discussion, reflection, reaffirmation or rejection in a way that could not have been accomplished with a static text. Thus, interviewing provided a powerful opportunity to explore each discursive statement I identified from the literature "in the exact specificity of its occurrence" and further to ask interviewees to help me "determine its conditions of existence, fix at least its limits, establish its correlations with other statements that may be connected with it, and show what other forms of statement it excludes" (Foucault, 1969/1972, pp. 27-28).

I conducted in-depth interviews using the method described by Kvale (1996). Initially 10 participants were identified and the group of participants was then broadened by a "snowball" technique in which further interviewing was based on referrals from initial informants (Schostak, 2002). For example, each initially-interviewed individual was asked to provide the names of two people who might agree to be interviewed: one who had a similar or convergent view to his or her own, and one who had an opposite or different view. This method helped to gather the names of participants who represented different key perspectives regarding OSCEs.

I conducted a total of 25 interviews. Potential participants were contacted by email or phone and were sent a description of the project and a consent form. No one approached for participation declined to be interviewed. All interviews were face-to-face and of about one hour in length. All were audio-recorded with the participant's permission and extensive notes were made during all interviews. Participants were given the opportunity to decline to answer any question at any time. Findings from the literature analysis and from previous interviews informed the creation and organization of the interview questions.

All interview tapes (both the actual recorded transcripts, and the dictated tapes of notes made during the interviews) were transcribed and analyzed in order to identify major discourses using the model of "meaning condensation" described by Kvale (1996). Using this method, transcripts were read recursively and identifiable sections were assigned a condensed meaning. In this way, many pages of transcripts were reduced to a more manageable number of statements and themes. The goal was to condense the data to allow analysis and synthesis, without resorting to methods anchored more in a positivist paradigm such as using computer software to count instances and frequencies of certain codes.

For most interviews, two forms of transcript were available -- the actual recorded interview and the field notes made during the interview. The latter were particularly useful for double checking material in the audiotapes of the interview, and in a few cases where technical recording or transcribing difficulties rendered part or all of a tape uninterpretable, they served as the primary source of data from the interview.

3.33   Institutions

Foucault wrote that, "[w]e must also describe the institutional *sites* from which the discoursing subject makes his discourse, and from which this discourse derives its legitimate source and point of application" (Foucault, 1969/1972, p. 51). In *Birth of the Clinic*, for example, Foucault focused on the hospital, the laboratory and the library. For sites more abstract than an actual building, Foucault used the term "surfaces of emergence". These included such discursive sites as "the family" or "the court system". The various discourses associated with OSCEs also have arisen from different institutions. I visited a number of medical schools, testing centres and medical education and certification organizations. In each case, I gathered as much information as possible about the organization and its use of the performance-based assessment. Sources of data included:

1. Interviews with key figures;
2. Institutional websites including mission statements, institutional activities and descriptions of the use of performance-based examinations;
3. Visits to testing centres where OSCEs and other performance-based tests take place;
4. Visits to clinical learning centres and standardized patient programs.

Analysis of data from institutional visits took several forms. I kept detailed field notes about my observations, experiences and interactions. As well, interviewing several key figures at each institution allowed me to compare and contrast their perspectives and roles related to the OSCE and its use at each institution.

3.4   Ethical Issues

This research was reviewed and received ethics approval by the University of Toronto Research Ethics Board in May 2004, and was renewed in May 2005 and May 2006.

The issues of privacy and confidentiality were considered at great length prior to beginning this research. Because the number of key informants in the field of OSCEs is limited, it seemed that attempts to anonymize the data would be artificial, and

58

perhaps might imply a level of confidentiality that would be impossible to achieve in practice. I elected, therefore, to state at the outset that the collection and reporting of data would *not* be anonymous. This was consistent with a historical research approach that aimed to explore the role and opinions of key actors who have contributed to the development of a field. The University of Toronto Research Ethics Board agreed. The consent forms clearly outlined the non-anonymous nature of the study.

In the presentation of the research data, however, I have taken a mixed approach to identifying words and actions of participants. In many cases, the names, dates and activities of participants appear with no attempt to disguise participants' identity. However, embarrassing disclosures which might potentially cause academic, personal or employment problems for participants were omitted. Participants shared generously of their time, their views and their personal affairs, and made many such disclosures despite their awareness of the non-anonymous nature of the study. To protect their privacy, in some areas I made the source of a quote or action anonymous.

Because I have worked and written about OSCEs and performance-based assessment myself, I know or am known to most of the participants. I grappled with the potential for conflicts of interest in two ways. First, participants were clearly informed in the consent form that they could withdraw at any time if they became uncomfortable with any aspect of the interview or collection of data. None did. Second, I built in a reflective element in the data gathering process. There are certain advantages of having an insider role, in terms of having access to key institutions and individuals and in that being known to participants can facilitate interviewing. At the same time, it has been is important to consider the degree to which my own experiences coloured the collection and interpretation of data (as it would in any research undertaken by any researcher). Thus, throughout the data collection phase, I documented my reflections and reactions to my experiences and to the information I was collecting. This material is presented in sections of several chapters and is intended to render me visible in the same way that this work renders the other study participants visible. The goal is to make more explicit my perspectives and experiences and to see these in light of the theoretical formulations I present in this thesis. It also provides an opportunity for readers to draw their own conclusions about how the filter of my own experiences and perceptions relate to the data collection, analysis and conclusions.

CHAPTER 4: IDENTIFYING DISCOURSES USING THE OSCE ARCHIVE

4.0   Introduction

Foucauldian genealogical research is not conducted by collecting all of the 'data' in a first stage and then moving to a second 'analysis phase', during which no more data is collected, and all of that which has been gathered is re-assembled into a set of 'results'. These are categories and procedures taken from experimentalism. Rather, genealogical research is iterative: data collection continues throughout the research project -- right to the last minute of synthesis, and analysis begins from the moment of the first interview. The research however, does progress in stages and this chapter presents the sequence that I followed: 1. re-reading the unitary history of the OSCE to detect discontinuities and thresholds; 2. searching for recurrent statements, subjective positions and sites of discourse (surfaces of emergence); and 3. outlining of discursive formations.

4.1   Re-reading OSCE Histories: Discontinuities and Historical Timelines

Beneath the great continuities of thought, beneath the solid, homogeneous manifestations of a single mind or of a collective mentality, beneath the stubborn development of a science striving to exist and to reach completion at the very outset, beneath the persistence of a particular genre, form, discipline, or theoretical activity, one is now trying to detect the incidence of interruptions (Foucault, 1969/1972, p. 4).

The classic 'total OSCE history' that is often told, and that forms the basis for most of the articles I discussed in Chapter 1, can be thought of as *a timeline*. Both the use of the article *"a"* and the metaphor of time as a *line,* underscore the idea of a unitary, total history. To begin my research what I needed to do was to try to pull apart that apparently unified history. As Foucault wrote, "the history of a concept is not wholly and entirely that of its progressive refinement, its continuously increasing rationality, its abstract gradient, but that of various fields of constitution and validity, that of its successive rules of use, that of the many theoretical contexts in which it developed and matured" (Foucault, 1969/1972, p. 4). As a result of re-reading, new patterns of "regularities" in discursive statements, arguments, and the rules that govern the repetition of 'facts', should emerge (Foucault, 1969/1972, p. 25; Gutting, 1989, p.

230). Thus the next step in my research was to re-read the historical timeline and look for events ("singularities" or "irruptions") that might signal breaks ("discontinuities") and shifts ("thresholds") in the unified timeline.

As I have already noted, Foucault placed great emphasis on the importance of "discontinuities" as a tool in the search for discursive formations. He said, "the notion of discontinuity assumes a major role in the historical disciplines". While in more traditional, unitary histories, authors seek to dispense with inconvenient breaks in the linear, historical narrative caused by accidents, initiatives, discoveries and other "irruptions", Foucault suggested that these phenomena were actually the most important elements of historical analysis (Foucault, 1969/1972, p. 8). Rather than being a disruption in an otherwise clean trajectory, Foucault viewed discontinuities as sign posts for changes in discourse. After a discontinuity occurs (signalling a shift in the dominant "regime of truth"), the statements that are commonly made are different, the subject roles available for individuals to occupy change and the new arguments are used to explain and legitimate what is 'true' and what is 'known'.

My search for discontinuities began with the small set of papers that I mentioned in Chapter 2, which presented the history of the OSCE (Miller, 1990; Wallace, 1997; and Clark, 2000). I read these several times, searching for evidence of shifts in practice, changes in tone or language, pivotal events or any other developments that the authors noted, or that I could detect in their text, that might represent historical discontinuities. Several appeared very quickly.

The first fairly obvious discontinuity was the emergence of the OSCE itself. Clark and others at Dundee tended to begin the historical timeline with Harden's invention of the OSCE as a sort of 'time-zero'. On the other hand, those in America such as Wallace tended to characterize the key event as Barrow's invention of simulated patients 10 years earlier. Miller presented these two events as part of the same shift, from competence-as-knowledge to competence-as-performance (Miller, 1990). Indeed, before 1964, there was little talk of performance. Afterward, the literature was full of references to methods of simulation and the performance of skills. The OSCE added to this the structure of multiple observations, but left relatively unchanged the idea of performance-based assessment. I decided to work temporarily with the idea

61

that both simulated patients and the OSCE were discursive objects made possible by a new and emerging discourse of performance. I marked this discontinuity as the period of 1964-1975, during which time there was evidence of a massive shift from testing of knowledge to testing of performance.

The second discontinuity first appeared to me in Wallace's history (Wallace, 1997). She noted that in about 1980, the term "standardized patient" completely replaced all the other terms (such as programmed patient, simulated patient, professional patient, patient educator, teaching associate, surrogate patients, etc.) that had been in use since the 1960s. She said this occurred when "the focus of medical education research using simulated patients turned sharply toward research in clinical performance evaluation" (Wallace, 1997, p. 1). I scanned a large number of papers published after 1985 and found that she was correct. With very few exceptions, only the term "standardized patients" appeared. She was also correct that most articles had a clear research focus, and I noted a whole new set of language imported from experimental psychology and measurement. I marked this discontinuity, appearing at the beginning of the 1980s, as the emergence of a psychometrics.

I discovered the third discontinuity while reading Clark's analysis of the Dundee OSCE (Clark, 2000). From the outset I found the language of his work to be very different from earlier histories I had read, with its references to "line management" and "chains of command" and "economic and human resource consideration". What struck me was the importance that he placed on what he saw as a huge "shift" in the use of the OSCE at Dundee as a result of the General Medical Council (1993) report, "Tomorrow's Doctors". He saw this as leading to "fundamental changes in the way the medical curriculum was to be delivered", and two particular developments. The first was a shift in administrative governance resulting in a migration of control from individual departments to a more powerful, central medical school office. Second, he noted that the OSCE was no longer administered locally, but in a new 'Clinical Skills Centre" built for this purpose. Searching more broadly in the literature, I discovered immediately that 1993 was also the year the huge national Medical Council of Canada OSCE had appeared, locating the responsibility for testing Canadian medical graduates, not with medical schools, but with an arms-length, central agency. One year later, the ECFMG in the United States created the same mechanism for testing all international medical graduates. It appeared that the birth of the "testing centre" and the changes in who did testing indeed constituted a discontinuity. Concurrent with this shift was another change in language and the importation of terms and concepts from business and management. I placed this discontinuity as beginning about 1993.

With these potential discontinuities in the OSCE historical timeline identified, the next step was to see if my preliminary observations about changes in language, roles for individuals and institutions involved would be borne out in a more extensive study of literature, individuals and institutions. At this point I turned to gathering information from many sources.

4.2   Recurrent Statements, Subjective Positions and Sites of Discourse

Having identified three possible breaks in OSCE history, the next step was to look for and characterize discursive features that might be associated with each of these strands of OSCE history, in an attempt to see if "surface effects" of distinct discourses were detectable. Before describing what I did, I will review briefly key points regarding Foucault's approach to discourse analysis.

In the *Archaeology of Knowledge*, Foucault (1969/1972) outlined the four elements that make up what he called a "discursive formation" (or simply a "discourse"). As I have noted, each discursive formation has four elements: discursive objects, statements (enunciative modalities), concepts, and strategies (thematic choices or theories). He used this rubric to structure many of his works, including *Madness and Civilization, Discipline and Punish, The Birth of the Clinic, The Order of Things* and *The History of Sexuality*. It is helpful to take examples from Foucault's work to illustrate the meaning of these terms and show how I have used them.

A "discursive object" is the product of a discursive formation and can be either material or conceptual. The object is made possible by the discursive formation. For example, in *Madness and Civilization,* Foucault showed how a discourse of psychiatry made various diagnostic taxonomies of mental illness possible as well as the more material object, the mental institution. Similarly, in *Discipline and Punish,* he showed how a discourse of penality created the modern prison.

A discursive "statement" (or "enunciate modality") is an entity or form of expression that is made possible by the discourse to which it is linked. Statements may be actual linguistic formations such as written or spoken phrases, but they need not be. A statement might be a numerical formula or a graphic representation. Foucault's many genealogies are characterized by his attention to statements, and in particular to the repetition of statements, for he saw the latter as particularly important in identifying the presence of a discursive formation. He took great care to elaborate the rules for the formation of and repetition of statements.

Discursive "concepts" are the systems or networks of rules that govern the use and deployment of discursive statements making it possible to say, think or illustrate some ideas but not others. For example, in *Madness and Civilization*, Foucault showed how a 20th century concept of madness-as-medical illness made it possible to make statements about the origin of madness that were not possible to make using the middle ages discourse of madness-as-spiritual possession or the eighteenth and nineteenth century discourse of madness-as-moral infirmity. By contrast, the discourses of spiritual possession or moral infirmity made possible statements that were no longer possible with the rise of a discourse of madness-as-medical illness.

Finally, discursive "strategies" (which he also called "trends", "thematic choices" and occasionally "theories") are the highest order category within a discursive formation. These can be recognized as epistemologies that organize the work of disciplines. Examples used in Foucault's work include grammar, epidemiology, psychology, natural science and economics among others. In the *Birth of the Clinic*, for example, Foucault showed how the conceptualization of whole populations as a target of study and intervention was linked to the emergence of epidemiological scientific theory. In *The Order of Things*, he showed that the theoretical areas of economics, natural science and grammar, were historically contingent discursive strategies rather than 'natural' or 'real' ways in which the universe is ordered.

4.3   Extracting Statements, Concepts and Strategies from the Archive

As I described in Chapter 3, I used three archival sources -- literature, interviews and institutional visits. In all three I looked for discursive objects, statements, concepts and strategies. I did this by using the discontinuities and thresholds described above to try to unravel the "total" OSCE history into different strands. In this case, these strands were not perfectly aligned such that one began as another ended. Indeed I did not expect this to be so, as that might lead back to a linear, progressivist, unitary history. Thus, I tried to characterize these historical strands by giving them their own trajectories in relation to the discontinuities identified above.

Table 3 helped me to organize information. In the first column I entered all of the repeated words and statements found during my analysis of the literature. Later, as I completed interviews and undertook visits to institutions, I added words and statements from the transcripts. As the table filled, I tried to synthesize an integrated discursive statement (called "example of new discursive statements") that represented as many as possible of the key words that could logically be put together. These prototypic statements served well as a guide to question participants in interviews about the degree to which they could see distinct discourses. Next, I placed the names of all the roles, subject positions, jobs and titles that I could identify in the literature, from interviews and from institutional visits into each of the historical strands. Finally, as shown in the table, I entered the names of institutions that appeared to be important in each of the historical strands as they appeared in literature, interviews and site visits.

4.31   Discursive Formations in OSCE Literature

I reviewed over 500 articles using the coding face sheet presented in Chapter 3 (Table 1). From each article, recurring words, metaphors and arguments were identified for the purpose of characterizing sets of discursive statements. Table 3 shows some of the recurring words, as well as a synthesis of how these words were typically assembled into statements, and a brief description of the appearance, trajectory and disappearance (where relevant) of such statements. It is important to note that, at any time, many statements were in use. Table 3 shows only a few examples of statements made. I will explore a much richer set of statements in Chapters 5 to 7. What I have presented here are distilled examples (one from each period of time) of statements commonly used. There were, of course, many other statements made, some directly resisting those which were dominant at any given time. The purpose of this first step of analysis was not to create an exhaustive catalogue of all statements, but to characterize some of the most frequent in order to detect patterns in the discourses. Contrary, discrepant and resistant discourses are also very important, and are addressed in chapters 5 to 7. It is necessary to first sketch out the primary, dominant discourses before it was possible to see what statements might be in opposition.

Table 3: Three Historical Discontinuities and the Associated Recurring Words, Discursive Statements, Subject Positions and Institutions: 1964-2006

Discontinuity: Objects, statements and subject positions related to *performance* **emerge** Example of new discursive statement: *Simulated patients and multi-station examinations (OSCEs) are new tools for teachers to more fairly assess the performance of students and to provide feedback to students to enhance their skills* Time period: Appeared in the early 1960s, was dominant until the 1980s. Still present and widely used, although less so over time.		
New recurring words: actor, model, simulated patient, programmed patient, patient instructors, new tools, teaching, feedback, student, performance, skills, OSCE, multiple observations, stations, tools for assessment, medical educators, fairness	New/expanded subject positions: simulated patients, programmed patients, patient instructors, professional patients, medical educators, medical teachers, innovators	New/expanded institutional roles: SPs first emerged at University of California and McMaster University. Patient instructors emerged in Arizona. Then both appeared in medical classrooms of various universities in the UK, US and Canada. OSCEs first emerged at Dundee University in Scotland and then emergent from medical schools in the UK, and later USA and Canada I visited: McMaster University, Canada, Dundee University, Scotland
Discontinuity: Objects, statements and subject positions related to *psychometrics* **emerge** Example of new discursive statements: *The OSCE is a measurement instrument for medical schools and testing organizations to reliably and validly assess the competence of candidates* Time period: Virtually absent until 1980 when became dominant. Still present, now sometimes criticized in recent literature, particularly European sources.		
New recurring words: reliability, validity, generalizability, data, psychometrician, candidate, generalizability, item-banking, standard setting, cut-points, standardization	New/expanded subject positions standardized patients, psychometricians	New/expanded institutional roles: Universities across North America (notably Toronto, Canada), Ontario Internationals Medical Graduate Program, National Conferences (Associate of American Medical Colleges (RIME,) Association for Medical Education in Europe (AMEE), Ottawa conferences), Macy Foundation Consortia, National Board of Medical Examiners (NBME), Medical Council of Canada (MCC) I visited: University of Toronto, The Medical Council of Canada and the Education Commission on Foreign Medical Graduates, AMEE, RIME and Ottawa Conferences

Discontinuity: Objects, statements and subject positions related to *production* emerge		
Example of new discursive statements: *The OSCE is useful as a tool for assessment of competence for certification and licensure, and for public accountability because it is standardized, efficient and cost effective.* Time period: Rare until the 1990s, rose rapidly in the mid-1990s and now dominant.		
New recurring words:		New/expanded institutional roles:
standards, competence, licensure, certification, efficiency, end-product, cost, cost analysis, investment, accountability, unannounced standardized patient, foreign medical graduate, international, global standards, international medical graduates, screening, language proficiency, rationale use, standard setting, expense	New/expanded subject positions: labour, employees, standardized patients, standardized patient trainers management, administration, operations, production	Testing organizations in Canada (MCC) and the USA (NBME, ECFMG), Institute for International Medical Education (IIME), World Federation for Medical Education (WFME), Association of SP Educators (ASPE) I visited: The Medical Council of Canada and the Education Commission on Foreign Medical Graduates/National Board of Medical Examiners. Association of Standardized Patient Educators

4.32   Discoursing Subjects and Subject Positions

As I noted above, participants selected for the initial interviews were those who appeared to be influential in medical education and assessment. Their names appeared in widely cited articles about OSCEs. These participants included Ronald Harden (Dundee, Scotland), Howard Barrows (Hamilton, Canada), Robyn Tamblyn (Montreal, Canada) Paul Grand'Maison (Sherbrooke, Canada), Geoff Norman (Hamilton, Canada), Gayle Gliva-McConvey (West Virginia, USA), Sydney Smee (Ottawa, Canada), Richard Reznick (Toronto, Canada), Gerry Whelan (Philadelphia USA), Paula Stillman (Delaware, USA) and Danny Klass (US/Canada). Appendix B shows the full set of participants interviewed as well as their current location, institutional affiliation, academic degree(s) and important relationships with me personally.

I interviewed a total of 25 people between January 2005 and September 2006. Twelve were women and thirteen men. Thirteen had a medical degree, six a PhD and six a Masters degree. Twelve resided in Canada (in Toronto, Montreal, Hamilton and Ottawa); eight were resident in the United States, (in New York, San Diego, Philadelphia, West Virginia and Delaware) and five lived in the United Kingdom (all in Dundee Scotland). Their roles spanned a wide range including: students, simulated patients, directors of standardized patients programs, physician-teachers, directors of medical educational centres, medical education researchers, psychometricians and employees of testing organizations. The middle column of Table 3 provides a synthesis of some of the key subject positions made possible in relation to the emergent discursive statements that I presented above. It is difficult to link the individual participants to any one subject position, because, as might be expected, most have moved through different positions over their careers as various discourses have come and gone. In fact, their uptake of new roles and language was one of the most useful sources of data about the rise and fall of different discourses and the legitimacy conferred on those who adopted them. For example, a few who were simulated patients in the 1970s became psychometricians, while other became administrators. Some who were clinical teachers in the 1980s became medical corporate managers in the 1990s. Thus I have indicated the major types of subject positions, but have not associated particular individuals with each role. This will be done in chapters 5 to 7.

4.33   Discoursing Institutions/Surfaces of Emergence

From the list of institutions that were identified as central to the various strands of OSCE history, I selected a sub-set for site visits. Five key institutions were visited because of their importance in the adoption of and promotion of OSCEs related to different of these strands of history. The University of Dundee, Scotland (where the OSCE was 'born') and McMaster University in Hamilton, Canada (where the greatest growth and development of simulated patients first took place), appeared to be central in the initial promotion of simulation and assessment of performance. The University of Toronto (where much of the work on large scale OSCEs and psychometric analysis occurred) appeared in many publications related to psychometric properties of OSCE and employed a concentration of individuals doing OSCE psychometric research. The Education Commission for Foreign Medical Graduates in Philadelphia (the first centre to create a large-scale OSCE) and the Medical Council of Canada (the first organization to create a national OSCE for all medical graduates) also produced much psychometric research, but then shifted to implementation of large-scale national OSCEs. Table 3 illustrates the main sites from which the discourses emerged and the subset of these sites that I visited in the course of this research.

4.4   The Outlines of Discursive Formations

One can identify a discursive formation "whenever between objects, types of statements, concepts, or thematic choices, one can define a regularity (an order, correlations, positions and functionings, transformations)" (Foucault, 1969/1972, p. 38). Table 3 illustrates that discursive objects, statements, concepts and theories taken from different strands in OSCE history can be logically grouped together as discursive formations or discourses. In addition to providing guidance for identifying discursive elements, Foucault also suggested the importance of sketching the conditions in which the elements (objects, statements, concepts, and thematic choices/theories) are subjected. He called these "rules of formation". According to Foucault, rules of formation are "conditions of existence (but also of coexistence,

70

maintenance, modification, and disappearance) in a given discursive division"
(Foucault, 1969/1972, p. 38). Foucault began his own genealogies at different levels
within discursive formations. In *Madness and Civilization*, for example, he began
with a curiosity about the discursive object 'madness' and sought to identify the
statements, concepts and strategies that made its existence possible, but radically
different in various eras. By contrast, in *The Birth of the Clinic*, he began with an
interest in a series of statements about the epidemiological and physiological nature of
human beings and worked toward an understanding of the related discursive objects
(hospitals, diagnostic laboratories), as well as the associated discursive concepts
(statistics, the clinico-pathological method) and strategies (epidemiology, diagnostic
medicine) that made such statements possible. In *The Order of Things* (1966/2002),
he was interested in deconstructing certain discursive concepts, such as the 'rules of
grammar' and the 'laws of economics' in order to illustrate how these were part of
coherent discursive systems containing and making possible discursive objects and
statements.

In my research, I began by thinking about the OSCE as both a material and a
conceptual *discursive object*. I assume that the existence of the discursive objective
OSCEs was made possible by different sets of discursive statements, concepts and
strategies (that is, by different discourses). As I have shown, my literature analysis,
interviews and institutional visits suggested the presence of three fairly circumscribed
discourses related to the adoption of and use of OSCEs. These three discourses
consisted of a whole range of statements, objects, subject positions and institutions
appearing in ways that suggested higher order concepts and strategic choices. The
three appeared to emerge and to be dominant during slightly different periods,
although I would not wish to suggest that there was a linear progression from one to
the next. Indeed, the three overlapped considerably in time. Use of all three continues
today.

The first discourse I called the *discourse of performance*. Although difficult to
pinpoint in its exact origin, its emergence and widespread uptake followed Barrow's
first descriptions of the use of simulated patients in his medical classroom and gained
momentum with the appearance of Harden's OSCE and Stillman's patient educators
and checklists. Many forms of performance-based assessment followed and created

roles for a whole set of new individuals in medical classrooms including simulated patients, programmed patients, patients instructors and gynaecological teaching associates. The focus was on a performance-feedback-performance loop and the behavioural modification of student skills. Chapter 5 is a detailed analysis of performance discourse, its origins, statements, concepts and associated institutions. It is a discourse that still exists, although one that has been partly eclipsed by the rise of the two following discourses.

The second discourse I called the *discourse of psychometrics*. Its origin was tied to a series of discursive shifts both in statements and in subject positions. The conversion of simulated patients to standardized patients and the appearance of a whole cadre of psychometricians in the mid 1980s created a very different group of discoursing subjects than had the performance discourse. These positions were made possible by a sharp change in the nature of statements away from the behaviourist performance discourse to one of measurement and the conversion of social processes to numbers. This discourse, associated with specific institutions, is highly prominent today, although, as I will show in Chapter 6, there is significant resistance to some of its tenets.

Finally, just over a decade ago, a third discourse that I have called the *discourse of production* came into sight. With statements and concepts derived from business and manufacturing, this discourse creates subject positions that are significantly different from the discourses of performance and of psychometrics. Linked to non-academic testing organizations with structures like corporations, the production discourse is in full bloom in North America. I analyze this discourse in Chapter 7.

CHAPTER 5: MILLER'S PYRAMID AND PERFORMANCE DISCOURSE

5. 0   Introduction

This chapter characterizes the nature of a discourse of performance, still active today, that began to have prominence in medical education in the 1960s. Linked to a movement away from knowledge-as-competence towards performance-as-competence, the performance discourse emphasizes observation and behavioural, rather than cognitive measures of human performance. Because of the strong emphasis on observation of performance and of skills, the performance discourse is also closely linked with methods of simulation. Key imperatives include creating methods of simulation to authentically represent 'real' situations, and creating measures of performance to capture desired competencies. As I will demonstrate, the rise of a performance discourse created and advanced in tandem with the evolution of new "subject positions". A desire for new methods of teaching and assessing performance created a role of for educational innovators and inventors. Their newly created methods involved human simulation and thus another new role -- that of simulated patient -- arose. The presence of inventors of performance-based methods and of simulated patients was made possible by the discourse of performance, while at the same time these "discoursing subjects" promulgated and extended the performance discourse themselves. In this chapter I first characterize the key words and concepts associated with performance discourse, then explore the subject positions within this discourse noting the gendered aspects, and third, examine the nature of institutions linked to the performance discourse. Finally, I examine some of the resistance to this discourse.

5.1   The Nature of Performance Discourse

'Performance' can be observed. In psychological terminology, performance belongs to behavioural aspects of human activity. Performance thus has less to do with cognitive processes and more with action, movement, speech and gesture. It includes approach and attitude. In the behaviourist tradition, performance can be learned or modified through practice, repetition and the iterative loop of performance-feedback-performance. Integral to the concept of performance is an observer or observers who many simply watch, or may critique or evaluate. Given the strong tie to practice, performance is often linked to methods of simulating reality because it is cumbersome or unreasonable to perform the same behaviours repeatedly in actual social situations. The goals

of those working in performance include shaping performances in desired directions and creating teaching and assessment methods to do this effectively. While performance is more familiar in the arts such as drama and dance, I will argue that it is also at the heart of a powerful discourse that has significant implications for how statements are made, subject positions created and institutions structured in medicine. Epistemologically, performance is linked to the performing arts, but also to early twentieth century schools of behaviourism and sociological concepts of the presentation of the self.

5.11 Miller's Pyramid

As noted earlier, among medical educators using a performance discourse, one of the most common references is made to Miller's Pyramid. George Miller created a simple schematic that would have resonance across the world of medical education in English-speaking countries until the present: a hierarchical pyramid of competencies. (See Figure 3) Miller argued that it was imperative that medical education move away from the assessment of knowledge only as a measure of competence ("knows"), and even beyond a testing methods that allowed students to demonstrate that they understood the actions they should take ("knows how"), to newer methods that could assess students' actual performances of clinical skills. He said, "Academic examinations fail to document what students will do when faced with a patient – to demonstrate not only that they know and know how, but can also show how they do it" (Miller, 1990, p. 64).

Figure 3: Miller's Pyramid

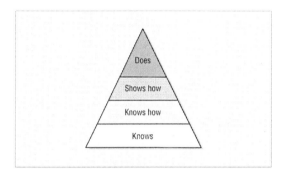

Miller argued that the ideal assessment of abilities would take place in real-world situations with patients ("shows how"), but that simulations could be used to approximate this ability. He also argued for greater use of assessment methods, such as OSCEs that require the student to demonstrate their skills ("shows"). For almost 30 years prior to Miller's presentation of his pyramid, the discourse in medical education and assessment had been shifting from an emphasis on "knowledge-as-competence" to "skills-as-competence". Norman, for example, called the period from 1975 to1985, "the golden age of skills" (Norman, 2005b). What is important about the appearance of Miller's pyramid in 1990 was not so much the idea that performance demonstrated medical competence -- there had long been a concept of the "art" of medicine. Miller positioned performance as the *central* competence. Foucault used the word "threshold" to identify the shift of a discourse from being one of many arguments, to being a dominant discourse or "regime of truth". In 1990, the widespread acceptance of Miller's formulation, at least in North America and the UK, signalled that such a threshold had been passed and that a dominant discourse of performance was firmly established. Miller crystallized this discourse with a simple graphic representation -- his hierarchical pyramid. Knowledge was still represented, but in Miller's formulation, knowledge was both below and subordinate to skills. Miller's pyramid had resonance with medical schools and medical educators around the world, and it still does today, as is illustrated by the many references to it in health professional assessment literature.

One of the moments that signalled a changing discourse from competence-as-knowledge to competence-as-performance was the publication of a paper by Gonnella (1979) that Danny Klass, currently at the College of Physicians and Surgeons of Ontario, summarized as follows: "Can you, if you know everything there is to know about urinary tract infections, do a paper and pencil test to see whether you can make a diagnosis or whether you could manage it? The answer is no". As in this example, the discourse of performance relegates conceptual knowledge to secondary consideration. Ronald Harden, inventor of the OSCE, illustrated this for me in a comparison of methods one might use for learning to tie one's shoelaces. "If it was a medical school in many places they would ask them to write an essay on the origin of the word shoelace, or give them a multiple choice question on the design of shoelaces or even ask them to describe the steps in tying a shoelace. Whereas really the only way of doing it is showing how you can tie a shoelace".

5.12 Key Words and Concepts Associated with Performance Discourse

As I presented in Chapter 4, a whole vocabulary emerged in the field of medical education in the 1960s related to performance and behavioural teaching and assessment. The term OSCE itself was one of the new 'words' that denoted a method associated with performance assessment. Largely the domain of a few educational inventors in the beginning, this discourse was gradually adopted by clinician teachers as well as the new 'simulated patients', who were increasingly part of medical teaching and assessment. Table 4 below reviews the key terms and concepts associated with the discourse of performance.

Table 4: Key Words, Concepts and Roles Related to Performance Discourse

---

Key words

Actor, model, simulated patient, programmed patient, patient instructors, new tools, teaching, feedback, student, performance, skills, OSCE, multiple observations, stations, tools for assessment, medical educators, fairness

Key concepts

Desire to observe the actual performance and behaviours of students in addition to (or later in place of) assessing their knowledge

Key arguments to support this discourse

Need to move from knowledge-as-competence to performance-as-competence

Improve teaching and learning via more feedback

Embed 'patient voice'

Improve patient care

Responsibility to the public

Key roles

Physician educators primarily

A small group of medical educators with PhDs emerged

SPs present but not empowered to participate in the discourse

.

Many changes in the medical education environment began in the 1970s in relation to the emerging discourse of performance. The most obvious of these on the pedagogical side was the decline in prominence of lectures and use of more interaction and experiential learning formats such as problem-based learning, earlier clinical placements and a whole host of simulated learning environments. As for assessment, the drive to assess students' actual ability to "show" their performance actually began with assessments on paper. Christine McGuire, a medical educator in the US, pioneered a form of written test called a Patient Management Problem (PMP). This format required students to synthesize clinical decisions related to paper "cases" and was purported to assess performance as well as just recall of knowledge (Harris & Simpson, 2005). Other formats of assessment that had been in existence for many years were looked on more favourably such as the so-called "anatomy bell ringer". This was a multi-station examination in which students rotated between "stations" in each of which an anatomical specimen with a pin indicating a specific structure was to be named by students. This examination, a fixture of medical school assessment, was confined to anatomy labs and histology exams (where rotations between microscope stations occurred) until Harden's OSCE extended the use of multi-station examinations to clinical assessment.

The literature that emerged following Harden's original description of the OSCE was clearly oriented to clinical settings and to the performance of skills. During the 30 or so years after 1975, authors with an orientation to performance continued to use certain key words and concepts. Given that performance was understood to mean 'what a physician does with a patient', it is not surprising that those initially writing about performance-based assessment were physicians. What Foucault has called the "medical gaze" in connection with the strong imperative of doctors to scrutinize patients in order to arrive at a diagnostic classification, was simply turned on the medical student (Hodges, 2004).

The link between the OSCE and the discourse of performance was evident in the earliest of Harden's writings. Indeed, many educators continue to think of the OSCE synonymously with the discourse of performance as represented by Miller's pyramid. Marjorie Davis, the successor to Ronald Harden as Director of the Centre for Medical Education in Dundee Scotland, wrote: "The main use of the OSCE, until now, has been as a robust framework within which to assess students' competence at the level of 'shows how' or simulation. It is unchallenged in its position as the assessment instrument at this level of Miller's pyramid" (Davis, 203, p. 255).

Anja Robb, Director of the Standardized Patient Program in Toronto, succinctly articulated the performance imperative: "When you are in a profession where you actually have to perform practical skills, for you to be ready to practice on your own, I believe somebody needs to observe you doing those at a level that's acceptable and safe and sanctioned by peers in your profession.... [Y]ou need to be able to perform". Danny Klass, a former Associate Dean from University of Manitoba, recalled that the move to performance-based assessment was essential because of the misleading way in which previous evaluations represented student abilities. In his words, "In the third and fourth year when the [medical] school was supposed to vouch for the students' abilities and the practical hands-on components of medicine, you would see the same individual rated as extremely good in one rotation and extremely bad in another. So I was casting around for a way to improve clinical evaluation".

Gayle Gliva-McConvey, Director of the Clinical Skills Centre in East Virginia, never met Ronald Harden, but speculated that his reason for creating the OSCE was that "rather than testing students on paper and pencil testing, they needed to have them demonstrate what they could do". This quote illustrates succinctly the core argument at the heart of the discourse of performance. There is an imperative to demonstrate behaviours, rather than knowledge. Said Gliva, the advantage of an OSCE is that "it forces them to demonstrate".

This North American interpretation is interesting, given the perspectives of Davis and Harden at Dundee. Both argued that in the UK, there was never a period when clinical assessment was not important. Davis told me, "I don't think you would find any UK medical schools depending on a Multiple Choice Questions (MCQ) examination. We always have had clinical exams – clinical aspects of medical training have always been considered important". Rather, as I shall discuss below, at Dundee the argument for moving to OSCEs was of fairness to students and of improving teaching and feedback (Davis, 2003). Davis said, "we may not have written about it, but certainly when I was a student in the 1960s and '70s, how one addressed a patient and the respect for the patient were taught and learned. This hasn't happened in other parts of the world.... [M]edical education in the UK has always emphasized clinical abilities".

Performance discourse partly justifies observation of students based on the need to "assure the public" that graduates are competent. Gayle Gliva-McConvey provided a commonly-articulated version of this argument: "I think that real patients' expectations are that communication is part of the relationship of the physician.... We have gone from 'my doctor told me so it must be right' to 'wait a second, I need to be empowered here and I need to have some relationship". So there is a movement from the public sector saying, 'I need to know if this guy is competent, who is going to assure me of that? I need to know if they are competent working with patients and not just getting an A on a multiple choice examination'".

The implications of this argument are two-fold. The first implication is that observation of students is necessary. The second, more nuanced, argument is that the 'real patient', who needs to be represented (empowered) in the education of physicians, will be represented by a simulated patient. Interestingly, there is very little discussion of the actual link between real and simulated patients other than in psychometric terms ('reliability' or 'fidelity'). Nor do these terms refer to the actual perspectives of 'real' patients about health care or medical education in any direct way.

Within the performance discourse, it is acknowledged that there is also a certain amount of role playing on the part of the student. In a reference that harkens back to Canadian sociologist Erving Goffman's (1959) book, *The Presentation of Self in Everyday Life*, Anja Robb noted that the function of the simulated patient is to get the medical student "into their role". She said the SP must have a certain amount of talent because "the better you play your role, the better the candidate will get into their role and display their doctorly skills".

Performance-based assessment has also functioned as a tool to help define and defend the medical profession's claim over certain areas of skill. Sean McAleer, a faculty member with a PhD at Dundee, drew a parallel between medical OSCEs and an OSCE recently created for the police in the UK. He told me that the police "were finding that a good lawyer could pass the sergeants exams, and it's not for good lawyers, it should be for someone who has the practical skills rather than just knowledge". Similarly, in medicine by the 1960s, with the growing access to medical knowledge that patients and other health professionals now had, medicine was pressured to define and examine specific behavioural skills that "belonged" to their jurisdiction. Common defences against the "poaching" of areas of practice by other health professions include professional and legislative measures that define exclusivity in certain domains of competence (Witz, 1992). Thus the codifications of behaviours that were central to medical practice and that "belonged" to the medical profession, were tied to performance, and operationalized by such techniques as the OSCE.

Validity is a term that appears in all three of the discourses that are identified here. However, what the term means within each is very different. In performance discourse, validity refers to the degree to which a simulation, be it for teaching or assessment, reflects 'real' clinical encounters. Key informants equated this concept of validity with the synonym, 'authenticity'. Demonstrating this form of validity requires evidence such as participant assurances that the scenario, OSCE station or other element seems 'real'.

The discourse of 'reality' in performance has resonance with acting. Howard Barrows, credited with inventing simulated patients (a development that I will discuss in detail shortly), noted that his approach to training simulated patients "is an approach that has been referred to often by actors and actresses as the method approach to acting". He elaborated that the core of this method is that the person being trained assume the role as closely as possible. He explained: "I would not say, 'the patient had this and that patient had that'. I would tell the actor, 'you have this and you have that'. After this I ask them to imagine this happening to them and ask them 'How would you feel if this happened to you?' " He said his goal was for them to "live the role". He would send the actors off to their homes or work to live the role for several days. During that time, they could think about what it would be like to be the patients with the problems involved in order that it be "a living, breathing sort of thing -- you don't want a wooden performance". Similarly, those who advocate the use of performance as a means of teaching or testing, place emphasis on the idea that

81

the simulated environment helps students to develop the behaviours and comportment that they will ultimately transfer to "the real world". In summary, performance-based examinations are expected to provide multiple samples of how they "would act" in "real clinical situations".

5.2   Subject Positions Created by Performance Discourse

The rise of a discourse of performance can be linked with the appearance of individuals called "innovators" or more often "inventors" by participants in my interviews. As medicine moved away from teaching and assessment that focused on conceptual knowledge, new means were required to focus on performance. During the 1960s and '70s, papers appeared in the medical education literature describing these new methods. The work of three people that I shall describe below is strongly linked with the emergence of the new discourse of performance. Each was important in crystallizing the emerging discourse of performance in both the pragmatic and the linguistic senses. Each spoke and wrote about the importance of assessing student performance, and each invented new techniques that could be used to operationalize the assessment of performance. These three were Ronald Harden, inventor of the OSCE; Howard Barrows, inventor of the first simulated patient which he called a "programmed patient"; and Paula Stillman, who introduced the use of "patient instructors" trained to assess students. Stillman is the most important figure in the introduction of behavioural ratings and checklists. These three remain widely cited today for the methods they developed. In addition to the subject position of "inventor" that the performance discourse fostered, the creation of a new role called "simulated patient" was a crucial development. Arising from Barrow's and Stillman's work in particular, but also Harden's OSCE, the role of a patient as a model or teacher in the classroom was not present prior to this era. Although individuals in this role or "subject position" were not particularly empowered to speak for themselves, their appearance was crucial for what they would become with the arrival of the psychometric discourse that will be explored in the next chapter.

5.21 The Simulated Patient

Howard Barrows told me during our interview, "If you believe in performance-based assessment, you need to have simulations". As I have pointed out, the invention of the subject position called "simulated patient" is widely attributed to Barrows, a professor of neurology who worked at the University of California, then McMaster University and finally the University of Southern Illinois (Wallace, 1997; Barrows 1971). Interestingly, the role played by the first actress described by Barrows was not one of a "simulated patient" but rather, "programmed patient". Dozens of articles in the literature make reference to Barrows' early work, and his work also appears in newspaper articles, published reports on medical education reform and his own papers and book. When I interviewed him at his home in Hamilton, Ontario, he was already well into retirement. Another source was a history written by Peggy Wallace (1997), a professor at the University of California (who began her career as a standardized patient). Her account of the development of standardized patients provided many interesting observations and quotes from her own interview with Howard Barrows.

5.211 Simulated Patients as a Technology for Teaching

Barrows framed his development of simulations, both in my interview and his interview with Wallace, as a response to the lack of observation and feedback that was part of medical education in the 1960s. His own teacher, David Seegal, a professor of medicine in New York where Barrows was training as a neurology resident, decried the lack of observational teaching. Barrows quoted him saying, "Nobody ever looks at medical students and how they're doing their clinical skills, or what they're doing. At theology schools they probably watch them give sermons and lawyers have their mock courts, but there is nothing in medicine". This formulation had an impact on Barrows, who would spend much of the rest of his career developing and promoting ways to build an observation of performance in to medical education. While his teacher Seegal addressed performance competence by observing students interview and examine patients, Barrows had another idea. After hearing a patient who had just volunteered for a neurological oral examination report that he had altered his physical findings because he did not like the student, Barrows realized that he might be able to train actors to present the clinical histories and physician findings. He did this first for a film and later for a live performance.

83

Barrows recalled: "I had somebody from the art school as a subject of the examination. This woman was learning a lot about the neurological examination and I thought maybe I could use her as a patient". Barrows explanation for this development is important. In his words, "The only advantage I had over Seegal was that I might be able to teach her to be the patient I want her to be, so I don't have to sit there and watch. And I would know all the findings and I would know the history". Here are the seeds of two important elements of the emerging performance discourse. Barrows' desire to have another figure (the "model herself") observing the student was a shift in traditional practices of teaching and learning. The new practice simultaneously increased observation of students and also began to shift the "labour" of teaching to non-physicians. But for Barrows, there was no intention of being less available in the classroom, as he described at length his commitment to being present for clinical teaching and feedback. Nevertheless, Barrows set a precedent that would eventually create the possibility of the simulated patients being the *only* teacher. The training of an actor also allowed the physician-teacher to completely control the role and its presentation, even when s/he was not present. This means of incorporating, while controlling the input of patients was necessary in Barrows' mind for the accurate portrayal of medical history and physical findings. Later in this research I will critique this control of patient presentations in terms of gender, ethno-racial and cultural dimensions, according to the perspectives and needs of physicians or others involved in simulated assessment. Thoughts about gender and race were not on Barrows' mind in 1964 when he sought to simply establish the idea that a physician could "train" a simulated patient (SP) to "properly portray her role". For him this was a significant shift in the construction of the role of the teacher, of the nature of the classroom and of the position of patients in that classroom.

Although Barrows did some early pilot work with simulated patients in New York as a resident, he really promoted the idea in earnest as part of his first faculty position at the University of Southern California. According to Barrows, students were very enthusiastic about this new form of simulation for teaching and learning. Faculty, however, proved to be more resistant. Wallace recounted the story of Barrow's invention, and made note of the objections that surfaced:

The father of this innovation in medical education and the most convincing herald in the history of the use of standardized patients is the neurologist and medical educator Howard S. Barrows, who gave birth to the first simulated patient in 1963 when he was teaching third-year neurology clerks at USC. It was not an auspicious beginning. In fact, for the whole of the time that Barrows taught at that institution, "No one at USC was even interested in using it.... Nobody was even interested in trying it." (Reference is to an interview Wallace conducted with Barrows in 1996). In those early days, Barrows was often invited to speak about neurological subjects, but frequently was requested **not** to talk about simulated patients. In fact, he was seen as doing something quite detrimental to medical education, maligning its dignity with actors (Wallace, 1997, p. 6).

Despite these early difficulties and in spite of negative medical coverage in articles that carried headlines such as, "Scantily clad models make life a little more interesting for USC medical students", Barrows persisted. He pushed on even though the USC Dean received complaints from medical schools all over the country (Wallace, 1997, p. 7). Barrows tried to convince the medical education world that his invention was a valuable addition to medical education. The legitimacy of this work grew a little with Barrows and Abrahamsons' (1964) publication of a paper entitled, "The Programmed Patient: A program for appraising student performance in clinical neurology" in the journal, *Medical Education*. And he personally wrote to every dean in North America who had complained.

Despite his efforts to spread his invention to other departments at University of Southern California, in my interview with him he said "it just wouldn't go -- I could predict how students were going to perform on subsequent rotations, but that didn't impress anybody". When he left USC, the program, in his words "collapsed". However, in his next position at the newly-emerging McMaster University Medical Centre in Hamilton, Ontario, it would be a completely different story. Barrows had spent time at McMaster in 1968-69 on sabbatical and "fell in love" with the new medical school, which was just being built. He found that his colleagues were very interested in simulated patients and said that he "had no trouble getting something going". McMaster allowed him to do many new things and very soon he was collaborating with Robyn Tamblyn and Gayle Gliva, both of whom would go on to be central figures in the development of OSCEs and SPs.

Barrows also met and said he was influenced by Geoff Norman, a psychometrician who introduced Barrows to studies on reasoning skills and to the use of quantitative research methods in education. Barrows noted that Norman was responsible for renaming the patients "standardized" rather than "simulated". (I discuss this in detail in the chapter on psychometric discourse.) Thus the wheels were set in motion for the reconceptualization of SPs in a psychometric frame while Barrows was at McMaster. However, the shift to a primary role for assessment and the full integration of SPs with OSCEs was not to take place until Barrows moved once again, this time to Southern Illinois University. At McMaster, he would continue to work mostly within a performance discourse that emphasized the iterative loop of performance-feedback-performance with the aim of improving clinical skills.

There is much less written about the motivations of SPs themselves to do the work. I learned more about this from my interviews than from the literature. Many of the individuals I interviewed who work as SPs explained that the reason they became involved was to try to improve the way physicians relate to patients. Diana Tabak, Associate Director of the SP program at the University of Toronto, told me that her interest in being an SP began after a visit to a specialist in 1989: "It was such a horrendous experience that I went back to my family doctor and said 'I don't care how great he is, don't send people to him and here is why'". Her family physician, who was a teacher and had worked with simulated patients, suggested she might like to find out more about the SP program. Now, more than 25 years later, she is a leader in that program.

On the other hand, Sydney Smee, one of the earliest standardized patients at McMaster University, recalled that there was often resistance from teachers. She told me that "a lot of physicians don't like the idea of fake patients. They see it as fake patients and [assume] you can't learn from fake patients". She experienced their dislike when a few tried to "break" her. In her words, "a number of times I had people go after me to take me apart, to prove the point that if they could make me break role, or make me look stupid, they could prove that standardized patients weren't worthwhile".

5.212 Actors and Prostitutes in the Classroom

It is useful to examine the nature of early objections to the presence of actors, and in particular, female actors, in the classroom. The newspaper articles written implied a sort of titillation of medical students, while the objections from medical educators and deans construed this activity as degrading to medical education. It is illuminating to note the words that were chosen by Barrows to describe the women who took part in these activities. They were called "models" and "tools" and he stressed the need for them to be "trained" and "programmed". Barrows wrote:

A young female professional art model with acting ability was sought and found. In the indoctrination program, the model reviewed a motion picture on the neurological exam as a basic orientation. Subsequently, a detailed neurological examination was performed on her, explaining each procedure and the basic terminology used. She was used for demonstrations of the normal neurological examination to medical students and resident physicians on many occasions. All this was deemed necessary in order to make her knowledgeable about what a complete neurological examination consists of and how it should be performed. (Barrows & Abrahamson, 1964, p. 803)

Others were experimenting with the use of live people as 'models' in the classroom. Paula Stillman (whose work I will discuss in more detail later), described using real people to supplement the teaching of anatomy on cadavers (Stillman, Ruggill & Sabers, 1978) noting that "the new teaching technique made anatomy seem more relevant to clinical medicine than using cadavers alone". She added that "live models were rated superior to using cadavers, especially in demonstrating superficial anatomical structures and landmarks". Another role for women in the medical classroom was as "gynaecological teaching associates" (Livingstone & Ostrow, 1978; Billings & Stoekle, 1977). The idea was for medical students to learn the female pelvic examination on live, conscious women (as opposed to a plastic model or on anesthetised women in the operating room, a practice deemed unethical and discontinued in the 1980s).

Perhaps it is easier to understand the early objections to Barrows' simulated patients when one reads carefully the earliest literature on such gynaecological teaching associates and discovers that they were often prostitutes. In his 1974 paper in the *Journal of Medical Education*, Godkins, Duffy, Greenwood and Stanhope wrote:

In 1973, 15 students were taught the pelvic examination utilizing two prostitutes as simulated patients. These patient simulators were introduced to the PA students as university hospital outpatients, and during the examination they provided the students with immediate feedback. Frequent comments included: "poor introduction", "too serious", "too rough" and "forgot to warm the speculum". The prostitutes served well as "university hospital outpatients" and seemed sincere in their interactions with the students (Godkins et al., 1974, p. 1175).

The article noted that the University of Washington Medical School also used prostitutes for gynaecological teaching. In both cases the authors noted that the use of prostitutes (who they called *patients* – in italics) was discontinued. In the case of the University of Washington, this was apparently the result of "a change in departmental policy and concern regarding the use of prostitutes" (Godkins et al., 1974, p. 1175). At the University of Oklahoma, however, there were other concerns:

In the authors' opinion the employment of prostitute patient simulators is not satisfactory. The prostitutes employed by the program were not articulate enough to provide the quality of feedback necessary for an optimal educational experience. Their employment was costly, at $25 per hour, and that expense prohibited their extensive and long-term use. Also, and more importantly, both prostitutes had abnormal findings on examination prior to utilization (Godkins et al., 1974, p. 1177).

Writing in a way that conveyed a sense of both accounting logic[3] and moral discomfort, the authors went on to explain that they replaced the prostitutes with graduate students, who, in addition to being sufficiently articulate to teach and free of disease, were happy to undertake the role for only $10 an hour As a result the medical school achieved both "a more controlled educational experience with improved cost effectiveness through a reduction in physician time" and saved patients from

---

[3] I use the term "accounting logic" in reference to a discourse about accountability and performance measurements as discussed by Broadbent and Laughlin (1997).

"repetitive, inept examinations by inexperienced students" (Godkins et al., 1974, p. 1177).

Not all schools started programs in this way. The University of Manitoba developed a gynaecological teaching program as well that Danny Klass, then Associate Dean, recalled had a decidedly politicized goal. He recalled that, "the women who did this, did it in a kind of missionary way for the feminist idea that they felt that nobody, especially a male physician, could teach this other than a woman who had experienced it". He described them as "activists" who "sacrificed" themselves for this teaching.

A long historical association between actresses and prostitutes as 'loose' women helps explain the attitude towards both in the medical classroom in the 1960s and '70s. However, even in more benign simulations, an uncomfortable attitude toward female standardized patients continued, albeit in a more subtle form. Sydney Smee recalled, "one physician…was so obsessed with how you only draped a certain amount – so little of the chest – that I started getting embarrassed in front of this group of people and I was starting to feel like a mannequin that he was demonstrating. It was the most bizarre thing and my only belief was that he was just so uptight about it he was just projecting it to the students and to me and I was picking up on all of it - that I should not be exposed at all -- but you had to expose a little bit. So, 'for the sake of learning we're all going to have to look at this'. But he was the faculty, he was the teacher, so, you know, I had to be silent in my role".

5.213 The SP as an Object

In these early days, the idea that these actresses might be teaching collaborators or even more radically, professionals in their own right, would have been unthinkable. Barrows' co-author, Stephen Abrahamson, was a PhD-trained educator in the Department of Medical Education Research at USC. The disparity between the authority and legitimacy of medical educators with a PhD and of simulated patients in the 1960s and 1970s was great. While the contribution of the physician Barrows, and the medical educator Abrahamson were recognized academically through named authorship, readers did not initially learn the identity of the standardized patient in

Barrows' article. It was not until 1997 when Wallace reported on her interview with Barrows that the world learned the woman's name (Rose McWilliams) and the name of the first patient she played (Patty Dugger). In fact, standardized patients in the early era were routinely referred to as objects, illustrating the degree to which they were conceptualized as tools for use rather than individuals. This objectification is at the heart of Foucault's concept of the "medical gaze". Barrows concluded one of his articles by highlighting the superiority of simulated patients over real patients, precisely because they lack individual personal characteristics. In his words:
While it is true that other techniques of measurement of clinical performance may be used similarly, the virtual elimination of the variable of the patient behaviour seems to make the use of the programmed patient a most effective evaluative tool (Barrows & Abrahamson, 1964, p. 805).

The link between simulated patients and the development of the OSCE was noted during many of my interviews. In most cases, the reference was to "standardized patients", a subject position strongly linked to the psychometric discourse that is a direct descendant of the "simulated patient". Richard Reznick, who led the creation of the first national medical licensure OSCE in Canada, noted that simulated patients and OSCEs are "so linked at the hip that it's hard to disarticulate them." And yet, in the early days of simulated patients, the focus was on teaching rather than testing. Reznick, for example, recalled that Barrows' initial contribution was primarily for teaching, positing that he may have used them for assessment "on a one-off level". Reznick argued rather, that "as the technology matured", the examination "became an enabling vehicle for the OSCE". This is theoretically interesting suggestion, because it separates the role of Barrows and other "inventors" of SPs from a larger movement that swept toward assessment.

Nevertheless, the link between the development of simulated patients and assessment appears in the very first paragraph of Barrows' first paper, where he made the argument that his invention was most important in its ability to advance assessment. Like Reznick, Barrows himself and others often argue in retrospect that the development of standardized patients responded to a desire to improve teaching, and to make up for the fact that most medical students were never observed interacting with patients. While teaching applications certainly appear in Barrows' articles, the opening paragraph of his first paper reads,

As in all phases of medical education, measurement of student performance is necessary to determine the effectiveness of teaching methods, to recognize individual student difficulties so that assistance may be offered and, lastly, to provide the basis for a reasonably satisfactory appraisal of student performance. However, evaluative procedure must be consistent with the goals of the particular educational experience. Difficulties occur in clinical clerkships because adequate testing in clinical teaching is beset by innumerable problems (Barrows & Abrahamson, 1964, p. 802).

This is perhaps one of the first written links between the use of simulations and the need for better examinations. The argument framed the paper and allowed Barrows to go on and make a case for the need for a standardized patient-based assessment to replace inadequate written and oral examinations. This same argument can be found over and over in hundreds of articles on performance-based assessment that have appeared over 30 years. Of course, it was almost a decade between the publication of Barrows' first paper and the article in which Ronald Harden described the multi-station OSCE. When that paper appeared, the utility of the OSCE was immediately obvious as a place for Barrows to use his simulated patients. Looking back over his work in 1993, Barrows claimed that the multi-station examination (he never liked the term OSCE) was *the* major development in the use of simulated patients in the last two decades of the 20th century (Barrows, 1993, p. 447).

Gayle Gliva, the first non-health professional Simulated Patient Trainer at McMaster, recalled that although Barrows was most interested in the teaching aspects of simulation, his thinking began to shift in the 1980s. He became interested in the more detailed aspects of student performance. She noted that this shift occurred while he was studying the clinical reasoning of physicians, work that he did collaboratively with Geoff Norman. It is likely that Barrows' shift to the more atomistic aspects of behaviour was influenced by the psychometric perspectives that Norman, trained originally as a nuclear physicist, brought to the partnership. Based on his comprehensive clinical teaching, Barrows began to move to OSCEs. Said Gliva, "we were trying to move from using standardized patients in teaching, into assessment.... [Barrows] was looking at the clinical reasoning of physicians...and wanted to move to where students would be able to do specific types of things, and so he got interested in the OSCE and having very small tasks to do".

It may be that Barrows' move to emphasize assessment in his speaking and writing about simulated patients related to his difficulties in securing acceptance for their use. At first, he said, the method of formalized observations appealed to his faculty colleagues because when it came time to give evaluations, they no longer had to circulate photos to remind the faculty who the student candidate was. According to Barrows, prior to instituting simulations in the 1960s, the faculty would sit around at the end of rotation meetings and say "Let me see that photograph? Oh yeah -- I remember that student. Magnificent -- really good student". Barrows explained that "magnificent" might mean that the student said "yes sir and no sir, Mr. Neurologist", which he identified as a problem. Barrows began to see that he would have more success promoting simulated patients to faculty colleagues if he labelled it as a means of improving assessment.

Barrows was routinely identified as a key figure in the creation of the new subject position of "simulated patient" whereby actors, usually women, played roles of patients. While in later years he was seen as a mentor to a subset of these women who went on to become the current leaders in a standardized patient professionalization project, in the early days, he wrote about them in an objectified, third-person way. He was always passionate in his writing and speaking about those he called simulated patients, but it was not until later that he began to think of them as colleagues in an academic sense. For example, in his 1993 reflections, he remarked that, "I have had many fascinating experiences with this tool over the last 30 years and I could go on for hours about them" (Barrows, 1993, p. 443).

Reznick noted that the SPs who moved into assessment progressed in their careers. In his words, "the OSCE certainly couldn't have developed without the standardized patient technology. The flip side is not necessarily true. What you had is very bright people...Robyn...Sydney.... You had smart people who wanted to do better and start something different and whose career has blossomed". Reznick went on to emphasize, however, that in his mind, this blossoming was associated with assessment, not teaching: "If you look at [our SP program budget], a lot of it is cost recovery from exams, right? Because the teaching enterprise doesn't pay a lot.... They have been adopted by the medical enterprise, but you could argue [that this was] because of their utility in standardized patient-based exams more than teaching".

As I have noted, Howard Barrows was an inventor who created a role for women in the medical classroom. Initially, they were passive models, used for exercises in performance. The role would change and evolve, but would not significantly empower the women themselves in terms of career advancement until the link to assessment began to create a profession for these women.

5.214 Non-Physicians in the Medical School Classroom

Throughout my discussions with the 'inventors' of simulated patients, there was a theme of gender relations. The fact that virtually all simulated patients were women was pointed out and Gayle Gliva-McConvey argued that this was so because women were both available and employable as volunteers or at low wages. A number of others I interviewed also commented that a large number of women entered the workforce at the end of the 1950s, and that they were readily available for low wages. Gliva-McConvey said that when the use of simulated patients was first demonstrated to physicians, they would say "you know, my secretary can train for that" or "I have a woman who could do this -- a coordinator, or my admin". As a result, the role "started to be a female one", she said, "it just became a very interesting phenomena that we were all women". Now president of a national association for standardized patients that I will discuss in greater detail later, Gliva-McConvey noted that even now, over 80 percent of SPs are women.

Although it would not be until the SPs started a movement to professionalize that greater legitimacy and power would accrue to women who worked as simulated patients, there is an interesting sidebar in the story. Around the same time that Barrows was creating the role of simulated patient, another physician and inventor interested in performance in the classroom created a related, but slight different system that gave SPs are more active role in teaching and assessment. Paula Stillman, an American paediatrician, was also a key figure in propelling the discourse of performance. She told me she was also motivated by a desire to improve the feedback given to medical students and residents. Like Barrows, she was distressed by the scant amount of time that faculty teachers spent observing the skills of their students. She encountered the idea of structured observation in the work of another paediatrician, Ray Helfer, who had developed a system for video-taping interviews and giving feedback based on short clips. She found this system of "interactional analysis" cumbersome, however, and invented something she believed would be more effective.

Working at the University of Arizona, Stillman first trained a group of mothers to give feedback to students on their interviews, using a process scale called the "Arizona Clinical Interview Rating Scale" (ACIR). Building on the positive experience, she then recruited an "extraordinarily bright group of people" who had chronic illnesses, who had retired early and who lived in Arizona. She worked with them to develop the ability to rate, not only general interviewing skills, but also the degree to which students took complete histories of problems in such areas as pulmonology, cardiology, rheumatology and neuro-muscular diseases. Finally, she expanded the role of the "patient instructors" even further to include physical examination teaching. She told me that the physical examination presented a problem, because to actually create a checklist for an external observer to use meant having hundreds of items related to each small part of each technique. Instead, she thought, "I could take two really smart people and train them on this long checklist, and get them to know what it felt like when each of these manoeuvres was done on themselves. [Then], if somebody was palpating the abdomen, they could say 'you're not palpating deeply enough' or 'you're exerting too much pressure over here'".

Sydney Smee, who worked with Stillman in the 1970s, recalled that Stillman's patient educators (including Smee) taught clinical skills and were authorized to give feedback on medical practice. Smee told me she would make comments such as, "'your stethoscope is facing backwards – you have to point it the other way if you really want to hear' ", and "'can you see the back of my eye? – why don't you take the scope and look again, because I can tell from where the light is that you probably can't see much' ". She contrasted the students' willingness to learn and to "appear clumsy" with patient educators to what happened when students worked with faculty members. Trying to hide their weaknesses when with Faculty members, the students would say "'yes, I can see the back of the eye' " when Smee's impression was that "they had no clue what they were looking at".

This approach to teaching, however, generated resistance in patriarchal medical schools. Like Barrows, Stillman found her work was not very well received. People called it "flaky" she said and "were very threatened because they thought it was only a physician's role to give feedback. In her words, they asked "how could lay people give feedback?'" It was this point, said Stillman, which led to her "whole original disagreement with Howard Barrows". Barrows, she said, was using simulated patients, "but he never let them give feedback" in the early days. They were bodies, and there was always a teacher in the room who gave feedback". She recalls that the first of these bodies were Sydney Smee, Gail Gliva-McConvey and Robyn Tamblyn. What they did was a silent but "extraordinary job with simulation".

Barrows agreed that Stillman's "great contribution was the patient teachers". He recalled being astounded when he observed a demonstration at a meeting. A patient said to a resident who had just taken a history, "What did you hear in the chest?" The resident's response was not what the patient was expecting, and so he took the stethoscope and helped the resident to hear the crackles in his lungs. Barrows reiterated: "He was teaching the resident how to interview and examine his particular condition. Paula Stillman wrote a paper on that and I think that's one of her great contributions – the patient teacher".

At first, Stillman didn't see the relevance to her work of Barrow's simulated patients. Her patient instructors were able to use their own "real" bodies and histories to teach and give feedback. However, that changed when she moved from Arizona to Massachusetts in 1982. Although hoping to replicate her Arizona program of patient instructors, she could not find a large group of retirees with chronic illnesses to work with her. She thus turned to simulation.

Stillman told me that, in the early 1980s, she was also becoming aware of the OSCE work done by Ronald Harden, and his "representative in North America", Ian Hart. Sydney Smee, however, couldn't recall ever hearing the word "OSCE" being used while she was working with Stillman in Massachusetts. Smee said "we would have people going from room to room, but it wasn't an OSCE. It was a station concept but we did not call it an OSCE". She went on to say that "it was a formative assessment[4]; the students would book themselves in. It was a circuit but it wasn't an OSCE". Smee noted that several features of this examination lead her, even now, to consider that this "circuit" of performance was not an OSCE. First of all, there were no marks assigned and so "none of the scoring issues where there". Next, it was the patient-instructors who were teaching and giving feedback. "We didn't use the word "standardized patient". It was "patient instructors because they taught". Smee noted that Stillman, Barrows and Harden were aware of each other's work and that they "sparred" from time to time. Stillman told me that she always believed that the most powerful use of the technologies of simulation was "formative assessment and constant feedback". She insisted that in her mind, "I don't think it was ever really meant to be used as a go-no-go [pass-fail] high-stakes examination".

Smee defined the differences among Barrows, Stillman and Harden as one of focus: "The whole concept – I mean the patients were teaching and [Stillman] didn't have Barrow's commitment to simulations. It was very interesting for the first while when I started working with her. I thought we were talking about the same thing. Howard [Barrows]…was very much into simulation and creating a patient for teaching, so then you worked with the faculty member [who was] the expert in small group teaching with a simulated patient. … And then I go and work for Paula [Stillman] where everything is on evaluation and checklist-driven and not a lot on simulation". . She went on to say that "it took a while before I started to appreciate how big the differences were [and see that it was the] same thing [with] different facets".

As I described, Paula Stillman was also working on checklists that became the foundation for OSCE measures that followed, and ultimately served as the raw materials for psychometricians. But Stillman was not a psychometrician, and while she later collaborated with individuals with psychometric training such as David Swanson, her own interest appeared to lie in capturing the clinical in a graphic form. As I have described in chapters 1 and 2, in the early days of performance-based assessment, the 'state of the art' in competency assessment was unstructured oral

---

[4] Formative evaluation refers to assessment for the purpose of providing feedback to learners, while summative evaluation refers to assessment for the purpose grading or making a pass-fail decision.

examinations. Using a behavioural checklist was unusual in the 1970s. Smee recalls that while "simulations certainly emphasized more of the clinical reality and the presentation, at the other end, [Stillman] had to train people and be sure that they could score accurately, that they understood checklists and they knew more clinically. Whereas, as a simulated patient they actually wanted me not to understand the problem".

Stillman's interest in checklists and ratings was not, at least initially, about mathematical calculations based on the data produced from performances. Evidence in support of this interpretation is that her data were not used for any summative marks. Rather, checklists were a vehicle to aid the patient instructors to do their jobs. Smee noted that Stillman was "very focused on having lay people as instructors". Digging deeper into the rationale for this, I discovered that Stillman articulated a strong commitment to the patients themselves and their role in having a place in their own care. In an article entitled the 'Use of trained mothers to teach interviewing skills to first-year medical students' (Stillman, Sabers & Redfield, 1976), she argued that mothers, with a little training, could be very effective in teaching interviewing skills and giving feedback to students. Further light is shed on this use of mothers for teaching in two later articles. In "Attitudes of paediatricians toward maternal employment", published in 1984 in the journal *Paediatrics*, she and her colleagues reported that while "most respondents were supportive of mothers working outside the home, bias against employed mothers does exist". She also wrote that "male paediatricians tended to hold more traditional attitudes toward maternal employment" (Heins, Stillman, Sabers & Mazzeo, 1983, p. 283). Stillman returned to her role of advocate for women and mothers as teachers in medical schools in a paper published in 1984 in the *Journal of the American Medical Women's Association* (Stillman 1984). Smee recalled that Stillman's "big push was to convince people that lay people could give feedback". She added that she also believed that "a student would confess to things if there wasn't a physician watching".

While Stillman was known to some as "the queen of the checklist", it can be argued that her use of checklists was initially for a very different purpose than their use in later years by psychometricians. The evidence suggests that her belief in the use of lay instructors and her advocacy for women and mothers as teachers was part of the rationale for checklists. They conferred legitimacy on these otherwise "non-traditional" teachers (Stillman, Ruggill, Rutala & Sabers, 1980). The whole process challenged the role of who was authorized to teach and who had a voice of authority in the medical classroom. Her work would produce strong resistance. In addition to patient instructors, Stillman also explored the use of health professionals other than physicians in the classroom including, nurses and nurse practitioners (Stillman, Levinson, Ruggill & Sabers, 1977; Stillman, Levinson, Navill & Ruggill, 1978; and Stillman, Ruggill, Rutala & Sabers, 1979). She continued to publish articles focussed on promoting non-physician teachers in the classroom until the early 1980s (Stillman, Burpeau-DiGregorio, Nicholson, Sabers & Stillman, 1983).

After 1980, Stillman began to collaborate with psychometricians (Stillman & Swanson, 1987; Woodward, Neufeld, Norman and Stillman, 1983), focusing on assessment rather than on teaching. She undertook studies looking at 'variables', 'reliability' and 'validity' and became involved in the assessment of international medical graduates (Stillman, Madigan, Thompson, Swanson, Julian, Regan et al., 1989). As I will show in the next chapter, these are all features associated with the new psychometric discourse that arose in the early 1980s. This shift in Stillman's work signalled a more general move away from performance discourse towards the positivist scientific and measurement orientation of psychometrics. Whereas in the late 1970s, Stillman published articles with colleagues using titles such as "The Nurse Practitioner as a Teacher of Physical Examination Skills" (1977), "Use of Trained Mothers to Teach Interviewing Skills to First-Year Medical Students" (1977) and "Collaborative Teaching Efforts Between a Medical and Nursing College" (1978), in the 1980s, her articles were entitled, "Assessing Clinical Skills of Residents with Standardized Patients" (1986) and "Is Test Security an Issue in a Multi-Station Clinical Assessment?" (1991). The "patient instructor" role that was oriented towards giving non-physicians health professionals and 'real' patients a place and a voice in the classroom, gradually disappeared in her articles and the writing adopted the new term "standardized patient". Whereas a 1980 article would discuss the role of "Patient instructors as teachers and evaluators", a paper published in 1987 would be called "Ensuring the clinical competence of medical school graduates through standardized patients".

These examples illustrate how subject positions create, and are created by, discourse. Paula Stillman's, like Howard Barrows', work was originally propelled by a need for inventions that would bring simulation and performance to life in the medical classroom. While Barrows did this by bringing models and actresses into the classroom and calling them "simulated patients", Stillman did this by creating roles for non-physician health professionals and teachers in the classroom as "patient instructors". These inventions both arose from, and propelled the discourse of performance as it related to simulation, clinical teaching and feedback based on an imperative for behavioural observation.

While all of this was ongoing, the experiences of simulated patients themselves were hardly documented. As a job almost completely taken up by women, the work was not well paid and often very hard. One participant recalled, "I used to carry home laundry. What man would take home a garbage bag full of dirty sheets and launder them and bring them back for the next exercise? What man would say 'oh no, you don't have an office, you don't have a locker to do your work' and carry around a bag and interview people in coffee shops and work in hospital waiting rooms to train them?" Getting the work done took priority and there was no thought that simulated patients would be writing academic articles and undertaking research. As is powerfully illustrated by Wallace's history of SPs, it was the inventors -- Barrows, Stillman and others whose names would be associated with the creation and evolution of this role. By the mid-1980s, the work of Stillman, Barrows and Harden began to converge. A growing interest in examination development would bring all of them together at the Medical Council of Canada and the Education Commission on Foreign Medical Graduates. And, with funding from the Macy Foundation, they worked to create large "consortia" of medical schools across the United States.

Not only would the new psychometric discourse affect prominent figures such as Barrows and Stillman, it would also have a profound effect on simulated patients. Academics such as Barrows and Stillman adopted the language and perspectives of psychometrics in their writing. In Foucauldian terms, this new discourse "flowed through" them and constrained and shifted what they spoke about and what they created. It did so for simulated patients as well. The power that the discourse of psychometrics conferred was different than the power that a discourse of performance conferred. Among the most significant implications of this change was the virtual disappearance of the terms "simulated patient" and "patient instructor" after the mid-1980s. In their place, the new term "standardized patient" appeared. Because of the constructive power of discourse, it was not just the names that changed. Rather, the names changed, because the subject positions and what they permitted changed as well. In the new psychometric discourse, the inventors would be replaced by psychometricians and the simulated patients and programmed patients by standardized patients. The roles played and the discourse promulgated by people would also change, and as the new subject roles demanded new ways of speaking and thinking, new competencies and new ways of using power, the individuals either adapted themselves (as did Barrows and Stillman) or the were displaced by others.

5.22   The OSCE is Born

As I have pointed out, Ronald Harden is widely cited as the inventor of the OSCE. His papers in 1975 and 1979 were the first to use the term in the medical education literature. But Harden was not alone in this work, and I interviewed some of the original group of his colleagues at Dundee. I will discuss the environment of Dundee in some detail later, but will first sketch out the nature of that first OSCE and Harden's own view of it. This is important because of the wide disparity in the way the interviewees in this study described and understood what it was that Harden had invented.

Harden trained as an endocrinologist and was working at the Royal Infirmary in Glasgow Scotland when he first developed his interest in medical education. Although an emerging thyroid researcher, and the first to elaborate the mechanism for the secretion of sweat iodine, Harden was encouraged by a supportive senior professor, Sir Edward Wayne, to develop academic work in medical education in addition to his research on thyroid diseases. He recalled that his original interest was in improving clinical examinations. At that time, in the mid-1960s, all medical schools in the UK were responsible for their own examinations. To this day there is no national medical examination for graduates of UK medical schools. Thus, one of Harden's first activities in medical education was to work on improving examinations. He was inventive from the start and told me about several early efforts.

He created a method of using a speaker on which the student could place a stethoscope to simulate auscultation of heart sounds, and later he used a model railway switching device for synchronizing audiotapes and visual images for self-directed learning. In his discussions with me, he continually emphasized the linking of his work with learning. For example, he commented "we thought we should apply new technologies and spur new ideas in facilitating learning". He saw improvements in methods of assessment as an extension of that goal.

A big change in Harden's career came in 1972 when he was recruited to Dundee University to address the problems identified during an accreditation of the medical school. The president of the university, an educational psychologist, was very motivated to recruit faculty with expertise in education who could address the concerns of the General Medical Council. Harden would spend the rest of his career developing Dundee as a leading international centre in medical education. Quite early, Harden's attention turned to assessment. He realized that assessment was one of the key drivers of institutional change. He had already begun to address assessment in Glasgow and had become secretary of the new UK Association for the Study of Medical Education (ASME). Harden noted that he was very influenced by the work of Professor John Stokes in London who was critical of clinical examinations (Stokes, 1973). According to Harden, Stokes called the clinical examination "the half-hour disaster"; Harden called it the "sacred cow of British Medicine". Harden, like Stokes, became critical of this system and used arguments related to fairness and subjectivity that would later form the basis of the psychometric discourse that I elaborate on in the next chapter. However, the 1970s were a period during which the UK and the US went in different directions. Harden characterized the concern that was acutely felt on both sides of the Atlantic: "You had to pass this clinical examination, but it was only one physician judging you and this was very unreliable. It didn't sample the areas of competencies and this was quite wrong". On the basis of this argument, the Americans went on to completely eliminate clinical examinations from national certification of physicians and until 2005 had only written assessments. The UK, on the other hand, retained their clinical examinations but experimented with modifications.

Harden was concerned with the issue of variability of grading among examiners (or what is sometimes called "subjectivity") in examinations. One of Harden's first published papers (Wilson, Lever, Harden & Robertson, 1969) was a collaborative effort that illustrated the degree to which a set of different physician raters gave disparate marks to similar student performances. The paper focused on the lack of fairness in assessment. Said Harden, "I found a huge discrepancy.... They were looking for different things. If a student was rather scruffy or had no tie, some examiners would mark them way down and others would ignore that and say it was the actual examination we're marking". Harden attributed to John Stokes a metaphor which is widely used today: the metaphor of examiners as "hawks" and "doves". Thus almost 40 years ago, determined to eliminate variability and unfairness in observational assessments, Harden set about to find a means to neutralize "subjectivity". Harden's first OSCE consisted of a series of "stations" of five to seven minutes each, during which students performed a specific task. Some of these involved taking a focussed history or performing a specific physical examination, interpreting a laboratory test or other task. In each room, one examiner observed and graded performance (Harden & Gleason, 1979).

Harden argued that "[w]e were saying that clinical competence had to be tested by watching the student perform and that we need to do a clinical examination". In this excerpt, and throughout his interview with me, Harden illustrated that, for him, the idea of assessment and observation of performance are inseparable. He strongly resisted a discourse of assessment that could eliminate performance in the service of psychometric or practical concerns. He wanted to avoid "what happened in the States where the emphasis was on the written and the notion that the clinical exam was too unreliable, logistically impossible and therefore the whole emphasis was on the written exam".

Harden said that rather than eliminating this problematic clinical examination, he was driven to create an examination that had three characteristics: first "clinical competence had to be tested by watching a student perform"; second, "it would involve a large number of examiners so it wouldn't be dependent on the hawk or the dove"; and third, "one would be looking at the process of what the student was doing". These features -- observation, partitioning of tasks, timed movement, standardized rating -- recall the "panopticon" example that Foucault used to illustrate the technologies of observation and control that began to characterize institutions such as prisons, mental hospitals, military academies and schools after the 19th century (Foucault, 1975/1995). Later I will explore the topographic structuring of observation in greater detail. For the moment, the important element is that Harden was the first to introduce these ideas to medicine.

5.221 OSCE Variations: The US versus the UK

After 1979, variations of the OSCE were taken up around the world. It is of interest that the way in which they were realized began to change in North America. Harden felt that there has been a misunderstanding in America on the nature of the OSCE that he described in 1975. During my interviews with North Americans, I found that one of the most frequently cited arguments for *not* using the term OSCE (in its association with Harden) was the concern that the OSCE did not emphasize interactions with patients. Dundee informants such as Marjorie Davis and Harden, on the other hand, said that the OSCE was never meant to consist exclusively of *standardized* patients (a new role created by the psychometric discourse that I will discuss in the next chapter). They both told me that the emphasis was most certainly placed on the "process of what the student was doing". Harden regretted that this fact has "gotten a little lost". He argued that "we used a mixture of real patients and some simulated patients -- at that time we called them simulated patients because these people train to simulate patients!"

One key informant I interviewed from the US told me that "Harden's version of it really had nothing to do with standardized patients and I was never a big fan of using the term OSCE". This informant explained that OSCE is a "very generic term" in which "anything can happen" and suggested that the term "standardized patient examination" was more useful than OSCE. Other North Americans also suggested to me that they viewed the "Harden OSCE" as having very little to do with patients. Harden noted that as far back as the 1970s "there was a huge gap in communication between the two sides of the Atlantic". At McMaster University in Hamilton, Norman agreed that, in the early 1980s North American and Europe "were two solitudes". He credited Canadian educator Ian Hart with bridging the gap and noted that the International Ottawa Conference brought together Harden and Hart as the vehicle that introduced the OSCE to North America. "The first Ottawa Conference was very OSCE-oriented and it was still a foreign concept to most of us from the other side of the pond", said Norman. Despite this bridging, however, I found evidence that a large gulf remains between the two sides of the Atlantic on this point. While North American medical educators certainly picked up the OSCE, Harden and others told me that the form it has taken is quite different from what originated in Dundee. In particular, the application of the OSCE to mass testing and the use of psychometrics to shape its nature and outcomes display a distinctly North American stamp. These developments will be further explored in the two chapters that follow on the discourses of psychometrics and production.

While the development of joint conferences and journals led to greater sharing of ideas, arguably those on both sides of the Atlantic today still share decidedly different perspectives on the OSCE. The US discourse of simulation has focused for decades on which forms of simulation would best tap into the competencies of performance, and has explored various technologies ranging from paper patient management problems to computer-based simulations. Harden, on the other hand, was clear that his objective was that "it had to be a clinical exam and not a written exam". For Harden, the discourse of performance is synonymous with a face-to-face interaction with a real person.

Harden cited, as evidence of success, the general uptake of OSCEs in fields other than medicine. He used the example of its adoption by the police in the UK: "I suppose if something is a useful concept, the test is that it is generalizable. The police are testing the same sort of competencies, communication skills, priority setting, decision making, examination -- whether it's a vehicle, a damaged tire in a police garage or a patient in the hospital, it's still the same principles. That they take this on board and use it is a measure of flexibility, I find very pleasing".

Much of Harden's work focussed on methods of assessment. Yet he constantly returned to the iterative performance-feedback-performance loop. He reminded me that his colleague, surgery professor Fergus Gleason, had created an OSCE that was completely formative; it was used on a weekly basis to help with learning by giving feedback to students. Harden was careful to emphasize that his OSCE was a joint creation with Gleason. While Gleason's name appeared on the first papers, he did not go on to such a prominent place in the world-wide dissemination of the OSCE. Gleason and Professors Woods and Preece, who I also interviewed at Dundee, were more concerned with the local development and administration of a test that they viewed primarily as a vehicle for improving teaching and learning. Only Harden set his sights on the more international scene and was soon speaking around the world about their invention. For inventors such as Harden, bringing performance to medical education was more a creative process than one of science and research. One informant observed that, "Ron Harden is phenomenally creative.... He keeps coming up with these neat things because he is a very divergent thinker, a very creative thinker who is no way bound by concerns of psychometrics. And I mean that in the most positive way".

A central observation is that for Harden, the OSCE has functioned as his invention and its promulgation was and is linked with his name and to his identity. Regardless of the changes and debates about the nature of specific OSCEs, almost all writing about OSCEs still start with a reference to him. Thus the rise of a discourse of performance opened a place for Harden, and for other inventors such as Barrows and Stillman to create, and to achieve a visibility that they might not have otherwise attained in their clinical work. Unlike the more anonymous role of psychometricians and administrators that I will explore in the next chapters, inventors were and are "named" charismatic figures, lauded or criticized personally for their contributions.

5.3   Institutions and Performance Discourse

Several institutions were identified as key in the elaboration and promulgation of a discourse of performance. Among these were McMaster University in Hamilton Ontario and Dundee University in Scotland. The institutions that promoted the discourse of performance were, not surprisingly, medical schools. In the following sections, I explore some of the conditions at McMaster and Dundee that created a fertile terrain for the elaboration of methods of performance-based teaching and assessment; spurred on inventors of performance-based methods; created roles for simulated patients and non-physician teachers; and promoted a discourse of performance around the world.

5.31 Dundee University and Promotion of the OSCE

5.311 The First OSCEs at Dundee

Given the central role of Ronald Harden in the development of the OSCE, it is germane to understand the nature of the Dundee context from the 1970s to the present. During two visits (August 2004 and February 2005), I interviewed six key figures, toured the educational facilities and met with students, education fellows and others at Dundee University and the Centre for Medical Education. In addition to Ronald Harden, I also met with Robert Wood and Paul Preece, two retired surgeons who were part of the team that implemented the first OSCE in the 1970s. Marjorie Davis, the current Director of the Centre for Medical Education, provided a longitudinal perspective, since she inherited her post from Ronald Harden. Jean Ker, the current Director of the Clinical Skills Centre, provided a sense of both her early experiences as a medical student who encountered Harden's OSCE and her current perspective as the coordinator of the clinical training and assessment, including OSCEs at Dundee. Sean McAleer is a faculty member at the Centre for Medical Education and a psychometrician who has worked with the Royal College of General Practitioners and the English police constabularies, both of which developed OSCEs.

As discussed above, Ronald Harden was influential in establishing at Dundee a place for the observation of student performance through examinations. It is important to note how he came to be at Dundee. In the early 1970s there had been a review of the Dundee medical school by the General Medical Council and, according to Marjorie Davis, "it didn't like what it saw, and told the Dean that something had to be done". It was at this point that Ronald Harden was recruited from Glasgow to reform the curriculum. As part of his reform, he changed the whole program of assessment. He also created the Centre for Medical Education, with funds from the Scottish Higher Education Funding Council. Both his new examination format and the work of the Centre took the whole university in a new direction. The new emphasis was on the teaching and observation of skills. Performance was to have a particularly central focus for the next generation of medical students at Dundee.

106

Harden's interest in assessment of performance and his early attempts with Fergus Gleason to create a new examination with multiple stations resonated with the Department of Surgery. Its members were enthusiastic about the OSCE. Robert Wood, a consultant surgeon also qualified as a physician, arrived from training in Chicago in 1976, and became involved with the support of the Chair, Professor Cushieri. Realizing that surgeons as a group would be against changing their examination traditions, he proposed a pilot test to compare the new OSCE to the usual examinations. Using a control group of medical students who had taken the traditional long and short case examinations, a group of students also took the new OSCE. According to those I interviewed, the results were convincing enough that the Chair supported the use of an OSCE for all students the next year. Harden noted that a number of political manoeuvres were necessary to initially establish the OSCE, including banning all the heads of departments from the assessment committee. This, together with other strategies, allowed a "quick quiet revolution" and a complete change of the methods used to assess students. A report on development of the surgical OSCE was one of a few publications to emerge from Dundee (Cushieri, Gleason, Harden and Woods, 1979).

From 1979 onward Paul Preece organized the OSCE for 20 years. He had joined Dundee in 1977 as a senior lecturer in general surgery, and had a university salary and an expectation to develop education. Although he had no experience with OSCEs or assessment, he remembers meeting with Harden, Woods and Cushieri. He found the idea of the OSCE "well described and rational". During the 20 years he was involved, his efforts to mount the OSCEs were time consuming, so that he did not undertake research or academic publications about OSCEs. He grappled with the slow adoption of OSCEs at Dundee. This included what he termed the "huge emotional trauma" when faculty experienced emotions with simulated patients for the first time, and the gradual reduction of station length from six minutes, to five to 4.5 and finally to 3.5 minutes as the number of students increased from 60 to 120 to 180.

Harden's OSCE, originally introduced in the Department of Surgery, was eventually picked up by other departments and used as a final assessment of competence for clerkship rotations. It was not until much later (about 1995) when these smaller, course-based OSCEs were merged together to create school-wide final examinations.

Dundee began to teach about their OSCE model around the world in countries such as Malaysia where Wood remembers providing workshops as soon as the early 1980s. He noted that "we are introducing it in all the international old colonies -- in India, Mumbai, Chennai, Delhi, in Kuwait, Saudi Arabia, Oman, Hong Kong, Singapore, Malaysia and Myanmar".

Harden also had a role in establishing a Clinical Skills Centre. He saw the imperative for performance as including, but not being restricted to, assessment. Final course assessment using an OSCE was to go hand-in-hand with opportunities to perform and learn during training. Like the OSCE, these learning experiences were also formalized and standardized, rather than being left to the vagaries of individual clinical rotations on the patient ward and clinics with supervisors. The pairing of a clinical skills teaching centre with clinical OSCE examinations characterizes the way the discourse of performance comes to life at medical schools. As I will show later, this is quite different from the way OSCEs are used in the psychometric and production discourses. In neither of these latter discourses does a clinical skills teaching centre play a role. In psychometric and production discourse, observation and OSCEs serve only assessment and classification purposes. Thus, it was instructive to explore the degree to which the performance discourse still existed in Dundee and to explore the views of those at Dundee about the emerging discourses of psychometrics and of production.

Jean Ker, who was director of clinical skills training and of the Dundee OSCEs at the time of my visit, located herself solidly within the performance discourse. Although there were some aspects of the discourse that she rejected (notably its separation of knowledge and skills that I will discuss below), the way in which she used the performance discourse illustrated for me that it is still very active at Dundee. Ker saw her primary responsibility as ensuring "that students are well rehearsed prior to going into the clinical arena for clinical practice". She described an iterative process whereby students learn skills in simulated settings, are observed, given feedback, practice and when competent, try their new skills (under observation) in a real clinical setting. She underscored the importance of more senior students returning from clinical settings to hone their skills in the simulated context. The key elements that make this part of the performance discourse are the strong emphasis on behavioural performance, observation, practice, repetition and application, with further observation. In particular, the word "rehearsed" links these statements to the performance discourse.

5.312 Views of the Limitations of OSCEs at Dundee

This ethos of clinical training that extends back to the origins of the clinical skills programs, according to Ker, infused Dundee thinking behind the development of OSCEs. However, she noted that very early on, there was a tendency for OSCEs to drift from the clinical learning process. Ker was among the informants that I interviewed who experienced OSCEs as a student. Her first exposure was during her medical studies at Manchester in about 1982. She recalled that the OSCE "just appeared", with no preparation and no link to teaching. "We were just faced with this exam, and we weren't prepared for it, weren't told anything about it. And between 30 and 40 percent of that year failed it". Both Ker and Harden see this application of an OSCE with no link to clinical training as being in conflict with the performance-based imperative. It is important to note the date of 1982 which corresponded with the emergence of the psychometric discourse related to OSCEs. Arguable the appearance of concepts such as reliability led to increased 'test security' (the effort to ensure that all examinations materials remain unknown to outsiders) which in turn helped sever the link between examinations and teaching. I will discuss this phenomenon in much greater depth below.

Ker described for me her strong attempts to keep psychometric discourse from overwhelming what she values in performance. She saw that for some, the OSCE has become "an assessment process rather than a clinical process" and that this causes conflicts. She feels that the OSCE itself can significantly distort performance if it becomes disconnected from clinical teaching. She argued, "if you've got a mindset and you've learned things according to checklists, then you can actually perform better in the OSCE than if you're beginning to develop those elaborated sort of networks in your brain that allow you to explore a lot of issues with a patient". She noted that Dundee tries to teach students to use "a patient centred approach" and to adapt checklists to reflect that. But, she noted, because stations are so short (four minutes in Dundee), in her words "a lot of our good clinical practice goes out the window when you are in an exam situation". She noted that students who take a more holistic approach "come into the station and try to do everything and they get really upset".

When I asked Ker about her views on whether the OSCE in particular contributes to effective medical learning because of it emphasis on performance, her view was mixed. She argued that "some people have used it as a way of learning" but it would be necessary to hold a particular view of learning to accept the use of OSCEs in learning. That view is one in which "you believe in [moving] from inexperience to expert" by "constructing things". That is, you believe that "you start off with a checklist and you rehearse and rehearse and rehearse it again [so] that you will develop a certain amount of competence". She told me that she does believe in the importance of practice and in observation. However she warned that the absence of reflection in structured OSCEs makes them less likely to result in learning: "I think it can also be detrimental in that, if you are thinking in 'checklists' all the time, it doesn't allow you to think, 'well why am I doing this?' So it can take out the why questions. I don't think OSCE encourages reflection". [5] Ker's second argument regarding problems of OSCE assessment related to learner self-direction and autonomy. She said, "I like the idea that you recognize what you know and then build on that and develop that further. ... I don't know if the OSCE really encourages that because the OSCE stops at the first bit -- are you able to identify what you know?"

Robert Woods concurred that there are limitations to the use of OSCEs and noted that he is fighting to prevent its use for residents at high levels of expertise. Yet there is a great deal of pressure to institutionalize such examinations. At that level, he conceded (echoing the literature I reviewed in Chapter 1 that criticized oral examinations), oral examinations "need fixing". But in terms of the use of OSCEs for final examinations for residents, he said, "I will resist this to the end of my days". He called his efforts a "war" with the Chair of a UK national committee that is attempting to implement OSCEs for residents at a national level. Said Woods, "I abhor its use for anything but medical students". What he rejected most strongly was the use of simulated patients.

---

[5] The centrality of reflection in learning a profession was a concept made popular for many physician-educators by the work of Donald Schon in his book *Educating the Reflective Practitioner* (1987).

On the other hand, he was quite pleased with the efforts of the Royal College of Surgeons to standardize questions and cases and to use multiple 'real' patients.

Ker gave several examples of ways in which she is trying to overcome what she sees as limitations in the technology of OSCEs. For example, she has developed "linked" stations in which one station after the next continues the same theme, or different aspects of the same patient problem, such as seeing family members, reviewing tests, and so on. Another invention was to create an OSCE that was not marked, that included group work and that built in reflection. She says to students "go away in your group and decide what you think are the important aspects of this examination - come up with a checklist" After 20 minutes she has them come back and discuss what they have developed and what they think is important. She said, "you find out what the gaps are and what they actually perceive as important. Then you show them your checklist and you say 'this is why I think these things are important'. That's about evaluating and about reflection". In this model there is an emphasis on observation, but the process also includes peer observation, self-observation and a great deal of discussion and reflection.

Important here is the way in which Ker pursued this discussion. She remained within a discourse of performance that included an imperative for learning, for feedback and for a link to clinical practice. This is quite unlike the psychometric and production discourses. These discourses often give little consideration to teaching and learning, and can preclude practices of peer and self-assessment and feedback because of 'test security' considerations. The following statement, made by Ker, is helpful in sketching the line between a discourse of performance (that emphasizes observation) and a discourse of psychometrics (which adds to observation an imperative for psychometric properties such as reliability). She said, "I'm hoping [the students] see the OSCE, not as a series of 28 stations, but as a series of patients where aspects of patient care and management and knowledge are assessed, so it gives them a more global thing to hang on to, rather than having 28 four-minute pieces of unconnected knowledge or applications". As I will illustrate in the next chapter, the discourse of psychometrics has been concerned precisely with establishing just such independence and equivalence of OSCE stations. Psychometric discourse also involves moving away from global measures toward atomistic measures of behaviour. In this process, the links to learning become disarticulated not unlike the discontinuity felt by Jean Ker in 1982 when the Manchester OSCE "dropped on our heads".

5.313 The OSCE as an International versus a Local Phenomenon in Teaching Practice

Marjorie Davis, current Director of the Centre for Medical Education in Dundee had a similarly strong orientation toward teaching, emphasizing that assessment is integrated with learning. We spoke about my observation that, although Dundee was the place where the OSCE originated, there were few publications that emerged from the Centre. She acknowledged this and noted that it has always been difficult for medical education to have credibility at Dundee. She told me that neither Paul Preece nor Robert Wood, originators of the OSCE, had gained much academic credit or career advancement as a result of their OSCE work. In an environment that valued research grants, OSCE development was not seen as very prestigious. Further, Davis noted that "this university will promote people on the basis of research, grant income and research papers published. Publishing papers on the OSCE just wasn't the same thing". Much later, Davis told me that at least 680 papers have been published on OSCEs, undoubtedly creating academic opportunities and promotions for their authors. Why didn't this happen at Dundee? The answer seems to be that the discourse of performance alone was not sufficiently interesting to granting agencies and journals. The discovery of psychometrics and heavily data-driven educational research and publishing, however, gained celebrity and advancement for authors. But this movement was not embraced at Dundee. Thus for reasons of resources, encouragement, time available and personal interest among Harden, Preece, Wood and others, a "data-driven OSCE publishing machine" never emerged at Dundee.

What did emerge was an international reputation for the Centre for Medical Education in Dundee, largely based on the OSCE. Sean McAleer felt that there was nothing particular about Dundee that lead to the OSCE. Rather, it was a development ripe for appearance and could have happened, for example, at Harvard. He attributed the uptake of the OSCE in Dundee to Ronald Harden himself, and noted that Harden's particular drive led the OSCE to be more well-known internationally than locally. "It's one of those things that has really dominated the world but in Dundee people just sort of accept it -- 'well it's there'". McAleer told me he is sure that Harden "knew

112

that the success of the centre was dependent on international connections and went out there and did the business".

Teaching, clinical education and innovation are core elements of the performance discourse not linked to grant capture, publication and other currencies of advancement. To stay within a discourse of performance that is linked to learning, feedback and the student experience, but which is not tied to psychometrics was to weaken the prominence and legitimacy of one's work. Contrasting the Dundee experience to other centres, it becomes evident how significantly power flows through the psychometric discourse. This helps explain why many medical educators in other places adopted psychometrics.

5.314 The Portfolio as Dundee's Successor to the OSCE

The discourse of performance continues to sustain itself at Dundee. It is not clear that the new generation shares Harden's passion for the OSCE, preferring innovations at the Centre for Medical Education. One noted that the map showing all the cities of the world where the OSCE was taken up, came down because "it got somewhat cluttered". Another said "that sort of pride in the OSCE when I first came to the Centre" has waned a little now that the OSCE is no longer an innovation, and because it did not result in the raft of studies and publications on its use that came from many other centres in the US and Canada. Instead, Dundee has continued to develop teachers (through its international programs for medical educators) and innovations. The current work that preoccupies Director Davis is the development of the portfolio for assessment. It is worth noting that her work on the portfolio and the discourse that supports it is an echo of the development of OSCEs at Dundee over 30 years before.

Davis also framed the portfolio in terms of Miller's pyramid. Whereas she described the OSCE as useful to assess the "shows" level of the pyramid, the portfolio, she insisted, can assess behaviour at the "does" level. In her words, "the portfolio has turned out to be a tool that can more readily assess attitudes and professionalism". With the OSCE, "we're assessing a range of competencies, we're thinking Miller's pyramid, we reach the 'shows how'. Whereas the portfolio is located at the level of 'does' at the peak of Miller's pyramid". Davis clearly believes that the portfolio,

113

traditionally used in domains such as art, but also in tenure reviews, is the next important innovation in medical education. She pointed to early portfolio uptake in places such as Maastricht (one of the early adopters of OSCEs) and in the United States. She even sees an application one day for physicians in practice. Following parallels with the OSCE, I asked about the degree to which work on portfolios has received attention in the literature and at conferences and to what degree this work could help advance the career of educators in Dundee. Her response: "There is going to be a big silence, while everybody sits down and works out what they can do with it". She noted that a very interesting version of the portfolio comes from Pat Sullivan in Texas: "She did generalizability studies. She looked at reliability of the postgraduate portfolio. It's published in *Advances in Health Sciences Education*". Davis went on to tell me how there were some early "unfortunate papers" showing poor inter-rater reliability that "threw doubts on the portfolio". But she is now optimistic that "there will be more studies coming about generalizability". Will portfolio rise and fall on the ability of it proponents to harness it to the psychometric discourse? Certainly this linking will not take place in Dundee. Marjorie Davis is an inventor and teacher using a performance discourse who may not appear in more than the initial papers on portfolios. On the other hand, others who are able to work within the psychometric discourse may adopt portfolios, create data-driven studies and gradually shift their use and construction on the basis of a psychometric perspective.

Ronald Harden expressed one regret about his career and the OSCE -- that he never got around to publishing much about it. Like Davis, he now worries about the future of the portfolio. Said Harden, "there is a big tension on the psychometric side still and I think there are very different views on this. Both camps speak very strongly. I see the same thing happening with portfolios. It's exactly the same as the OSCE story. It is measuring something that isn't easy to measure -- students taking responsibility for their own learning is one of the things. But the questions we are getting are the same. 'Is it reliable?' 'Is it too much logistics?' It is exactly the same scenario revisited".

At the end of her interview, Davis told me, "it's not rocket science, but with just a little bit of help we can help the teachers to give the students a very, very much better educational experience". A few weeks later, across the ocean at the National Board of Medical examiners in the US, another medical educator would tell me that the recent launch of the national OSCE for 25,000 medical graduates a year, was very much like rocket science and felt like "putting man on the moon".

5.315   Psychometric versus Performance Discourse at Dundee

Sean McAleer was trained as a psychologist and psychometrician, and I was very curious to understand his role at Dundee, in particular as psychometricians in other places, such as McMaster and the University of Toronto promoted the discourse related to OSCEs and assessment and pressed for a greater role for psychometrics. McAleer, like his colleagues in North America, was part of an influx of psychometricians into medical schools and testing organizations in the 1980s. But psychometric narrative is not dominant at Dundee and indeed it is looked on with some hostility. What is the role of a psychometrician in this environment? Although McAleer started his role with a keen interest in the psychometric aspects of assessment, having helped the Royal College of General Practitioners with their OSCE development, he began to shift his perspective at Dundee. Noting a concern with an overemphasis on reliability and measurement, and placing priority on the impact of learning, he has adopted the performance discourse similar to others I met at Dundee, more so than the psychometricians I met in North America. While conversant about issues of measurement and psychometrics, he told me he now prefers his work with graduate students and teaching. He is still involved in OSCEs, but his role has been one of faculty development about how to use OSCEs and improving their role in teaching and learning. He insisted that the presence of psychometricians like him helped advance the accountability and transparency of medical institutions; however, he argued that this can be accomplished by undertaking work that is educational as much as by working in the realm of highly analytic statistical analysis of examinations.

McAleer arrived in Dundee at the apex of the OSCE development and dissemination in the mid 1980s. Although he did some early work on statistics, today he is critical of the role of statistics and OSCEs. "Sometimes I think the problem of the statistic is that people put too much stock in it. They get caught up in the numbers and don't realize what's happening to the candidates and the people involved. Fifteen years ago, I would have thought reliability was the be-all and end-all. So you've got these very reliable exams, or they would be gong toward reliability, but what about the validity? People were saying, does this really happen in real life? They've got good stats to show that it's reliable, but it doesn't relate to what we're doing on the wards". McAleer called this a "reliability phase" that he believes has now passed. Cees van der Vleuten (2000) in the Netherlands is another psychometrician who has called for a pullback from too much emphasis on reliability. In the UK and the Netherlands the call is for a return to a more "authentic" environment where clinical teaching better reflects the practice environment and where continual, low-stakes assessment will lead to feedback. There is resistance to an overemphasis on reliability and checklists in North America as well, but there, the focus was not on dispensing with measures such as Cronbach's alpha[6], but rather using psychometric approaches to examine other instruments such as global ratings. The argument to stop using OSCEs (or not to start) for summative testing and for post-medical school graduates that has been made in the UK and Holland for several years is just emerging in Canada, but I did not hear it articulated during my interviews in the United States. McAleer illustrated the degree to which he is speaking from a discourse of performance, but not necessarily of psychometrics when he argued that large-scale examinations are not even necessary or desirable. "I am not a great believer in exams anyway. I think with a good formative assessment, you don't need exams. You don't need summative assessment".

5.32   McMaster University

5.321   The "Hippy Dippy Days" at McMaster

Given the important role McMaster University played in the history of simulated patients, I interviewed five key informants who worked in the past or who are currently employed there. I also visited their Department of Medical Education. My interviews included former faculty member Howard Barrows, current faculty member Geoff Norman, and previous members of the Simulated Patient Program, Gayle Gliva-McConvey, Sydney Smee and Robyn Tamblyn.

---

[6] Cronbach's alpha is a statistical measure of the reliability of a set of observations, such as different examination questions or OSCE stations. Cronbach's alpha is discussed at length in Chapter 6.

McMaster University Medical School was founded in 1966 and strove from the outset to change the culture of medical education. The traditional didactic curriculum gave way to problem-based learning, a type of learning characterized by simulated paper cases. Later, the first simulated patient program developed and, as noted above, it was at McMaster that Howard Barrows first found a supportive environment for his work in simulation that had been so roundly rejected while he was in California. Many key informants talked about the importance of McMaster, not only in its creation and acceptance of simulated patients, but also in its rejection of classical forms of testing and teaching. Sydney Smee recalled being a teenager during the "Hippie Dippy Days" at McMaster, characterized by an open and experimental environment in the '70s.

By all accounts, McMaster's initial adoption of many forms of simulation was in the service of education and learning, with relatively little emphasis on assessment[7]. Certainly there were assessments, but McMaster had broken sharply with the history of medical students assessment by eliminating all multiple choice question examinations from its curriculum. Even after its first class of graduates had an elevated failure rate on the national Medical Council of Canada multiple choice examinations, McMaster maintained its position that memorization of factual information was not associated with good medical practice nor lifelong learning. In an article published in 1976 and entitled "Medical student evaluation in the absence of examinations", Simpson argued that, "traditional examination systems achieve a high degree of pseudo-precision, producing relatively little information that is constructively useful for students or teachers, and conveying it in the form of scores and marks that appear falsely accurate". He went on to describe "the system currently being evolved in the McMaster University M.D. Programme" and its focus on self assessment rather than more traditional knowledge-based examinations (Simpson, 1976, p. 22).

---

[7] McMaster was, and remains, one of a group of medical schools that have features which distinguish them from "traditional" medical schools. These features include problem-based learning, a community orientation, early clinical exposure, few or no examinations and formative assessment methods to name a few. This group of medical schools also includes Maastricht University in Holland, Newcastle University in Australia and Linchoping University in Sweden, among others.

Geoff Norman, a member of faculty at McMaster since the 1970s, provided me with an overview of the history of McMaster that he had recently been studying. He argued that many of the inventions and values associated with McMaster were products of what he called "happenstance". While he did give credit to an environment that also spawned many "inventors", and noted that there was a certain discourse at McMaster that drew on ideas that were prominent in the 1960s, he argued that the "Founding Fathers" were not actually familiar with educational theory or methods. He saw them as merely stumbling on many of the then-radical developments such as problem-based-learning, the "non-expert tutor" and the elimination of lectures and examinations. In preparation for a new round of curriculum renewal, he had conducted a series of interviews with some of the original founders of the medical school and had learned that problem-based learning was inspired by the business school curriculum at Harvard. He also heard that the non-expert tutor was a solution invented for a couple of problematic faculty who dominated sessions with their own research. He also learned that the deletion of lectures occurred when a pragmatic dean needed to cut big chunks of curriculum time because the government approved a three-year rather than a four-year program. Said Norman, "in other words, all of them have more to do with the personalities and the happenstance -- the founding fathers were a bunch of pragmatic local guys who didn't know anything about John Dewey".

In terms of assessment there was certainly a different culture at McMaster than at other Canadian medical schools. Norman told me that "the founding fathers wanted to avoid the tyranny of multiple choice questions and standardized examinations and teaching to the test". He related this to an emerging critique in medical education of the problem of too many objectives constraining learning. There were two major results of this approach, according to Norman. The first was that individual tutors took on the most important role in student assessment. He noted that this was based on the Oxford-Cambridge model of the one-to-one tutor. But in his words, "we couldn't afford one-to-one so it was one-to-five". The second was the notion that there should be a periodic assessment for students that was not solely summative. Norman told me that the minutes of meetings from the 1960s document discussion about a progress test -- a test administered at regular intervals for the purpose of giving feedback to students. He paraphrased the documents as saying, "we see that there could be some value of multiple choice (MCQ) tests because of their good properties and their value for feedback to the students. But of course, the challenge would be to develop a test which does not get linked to the curriculum and is not used as a final examination". This description of a progress test would be much discussed in the medical education literature, and was implemented at Maastricht University in Holland in the 1990s. However, it would not be implemented at McMaster until the year 2005, suggesting that the rejection of MCQs in 1966 had considerable momentum.

While McMaster was rejecting traditional forms of assessment, the national licensure examination in Canada (LMCC) in the 1970s and 1980s was a multiple choice written test only (the OSCE was not added until 1995). A rising failure rate among the McMaster graduates on this test caused controversy about assessment practices. According to Norman, "the first class had a failure rate of zero, the second class had a failure rate of a few percent and the third class had a fairly high failure rate of 10 percent". A study done internally looked for a relationship between tutor evaluations and outcomes on the national examination and was unable to show one according to Norman. Although even a 10 percent failure rate concerned only five or six students, it sent shock waves throughout McMaster. Norman argued that this solidified a "dogma" against summative assessment. The MCC exam itself would be the object of criticism, not the failing students or the McMaster curriculum. Said Norman, "in those days you realized that this is not a curriculum, it is a religion. So objective assessment is bad and subjective assessment is good. In the sixties, we didn't want to grade people and rank people -- that's bad. So very rapidly, they adopted a dogma that tutor evaluation was necessary and sufficient despite evidence accruing that it wasn't".

At the time, Norman proposed a "reliability study of tutor evaluation" but resistance to having a ranking system for students to even perform such a study led to it never being carried out. At this time, at McMaster University, the discourse of psychometrics was not dominant. Even with the results of a national examination in hand, the dominant discourse at McMaster did not accommodate discussion of experimentation or of psychometric domains such as "reliability". Undeterred, Norman continued his research, noting that "I had to pay McMaster students to participate in my studies, because any kind of objective assessment was absolutely

119

ruled out of bounds. So they were all studies done peripheral to the curriculum where students were volunteers and they were paid as subjects".

At the same time, by all accounts, McMaster was developing a flourishing culture of performance. Barrow's simulated patient program was taking root and attention to student performance in groups became the norm. The development of skills was held in high regard by several individuals who much later would go on to be key figures in simulation, such as Gayle Gliva, Sydney Smee and Robyn Tamblyn who were working at McMaster and developing models of performance-based teaching and assessment. In summary, during the 1970s and into the 1980s, the performance discourse was dominant at McMaster.

5.322   McMaster's Reputation, Student Performance and Privileging the Psychometric

Officially McMaster's environment did not permit assessment consistent with a more quantitative psychometric discourse. This was understood to be an incompatibility between the development of "general problem solving ability", believed to be fostered by a problem-based curriculum, and the "regurgitation of facts" associated with the combination of didactic lecture and multiple-choice questions. Nevertheless, Norman pointed out to me that he continued to try to move assessment in a psychometric direction. He worked with his colleague Arthur Rothman, a psychometrician who had achieved a central place in the culture of assessment at the University of Toronto. In Norman's words, "I cut a deal with Arthur that in 1990, the class could write the 1989 test -- the one that had the 19% failure rate. Then we could say to individual students, 'you got 222, your chances of passing the LMCC based on last year's class was x percent'. So they got detailed feedback. In 1990, the failure rate was four percent". Thus, without changing anything at all at McMaster, students were able to enter into a parallel system of assessment based in Toronto that aligned them with the measurement priorities of the national examination. The psychometrics of testing, despite the 'dogma' against it at McMaster, came in through the back door. Norman concluded: "At that point, things started to change -- we got a whole new culture that was no longer based on religious dogma, it was based on evidence".

120

Perhaps because of the development of those parallel systems -- a performance culture officially sanctioned at McMaster and an unofficial psychometric culture borrowed from the University of Toronto -- simulation and testing were not as strongly linked at McMaster as they were at other schools. Richard Reznick noted that, despite Howard Barrows' work and the very strong association between standardized patients and OSCEs that would emerge in most places; this did not happen at McMaster. For example, faculty from McMaster were not involved in the early development of the Medical Council of Canada OSCE. Glenn Regehr, a faculty member at the University of Toronto, noted that rather than developing methods of assessment in the psychometric tradition, inventors such as Howard Barrows who found a fertile atmosphere for creativity at McMaster did not move into testing early on. He noted that the environment instead was evolved by "inventors -- very creative people who chose not to be restrained by typical things". But today, he noted, many of the inventors have left. He added that the growing influence of psychometricians and researchers have shifted the focus so that, in his words, McMaster will now have to be "creative within the confines of psychometrics". [8]

Speaking of the present, Norman told me that "everything has changed". He spoke of the new chair of admissions as "the ultimate empiricist". Contrasting this man's approach with that of previous years, Norman said, "He's generated more questions. I mean I just finished analyzing his question, 'What is the reliability of our grades?' We talk of GPA all the time. To what extent does a person's first year GPA correlate with their second year GPA? Answer: 0.8. The reliability of overall GPA across all four years is 0.96". Norman observed that it is now acceptable to ask such questions at McMaster. He explained that "there is legitimacy in asking these questions and now we have a culture where when somebody says 'let's do this', somebody else says 'where's the evidence'?" Participants in my interviews also reminded me that McMaster is considered the home of evidence-based medicine, where its inventor, quantitative psychometrician David Sackett, is located. And so, it would appear in 2006 that the discourse of evidence, of science and of objectivity that I have called the

---

[8] McMaster is adopting a "progress test" – a series of repeated multiple choice tests, administered every 3-6 months, drawn from a large bank of questions. The principle is that students' overall scores rise over time and that the pattern of scores can be used to monitor their progress.

discourse of psychometrics has overtaken that of performance at McMaster
University Faculty of Medicine.

5.323 McMaster versus Dundee

In summary, I found a very different trajectory for the performance and psychometric
discourses at McMaster University and Dundee University. While McMaster rejected
testing altogether in the 1970s, it has moved strongly in this direction now as part of a
greater legitimization of the psychometric discourse and a greater role for
psychometricians. Dundee, on the other hand, having invented the OSCE, more
strongly resisted the development of psychometric approaches. It has not created an
environment in which psychometricians have had nearly the same power to shift the
discourse.

Before turning to look at psychometric discourse in the next chapter, I will briefly
consider some of the key resistances that have been mounted against the performance
discourse.

5.4   Thresholds and Resistances

Foucault argued that historical events are "contingent" on shifts in discourse that
allow new phenomena to emerge. If he were interpreting the OSCE, he would have
placed less weight on Harden's invention of the OSCE, Stillman's invention of patient
instructors or Barrows' invention of SPs than my participants and more on
understanding the contingencies that allowed these to emerge. While Harden is
credited with coining the term OSCE and first describing its nature, it is clear that the
emergence of concepts of simulated patients and of standardized behavioural
measures paved the way for the 'discovery' of the OSCE. As Sydney Smee observed,
Barrows had to "convince people that you can use non-patients for teaching
purposes…[and] that you can train someone to replicate it" and second, Stillman had
to show that "[lay] people can give feedback and keep a fairly decent record with
accuracy". Once these two things had been accomplished, "then an OSCE became
possible, but you had to get past both of those things". By about 1980, the discourse
of performance was widespread and achieving dominance in medical education.

122

Publications in journals and presentations and international conference were focused on methods of teaching and assessment based on performance. Both the GPEP report[9] (Association of American Medical Colleges, 1984) and the Statement of the Consensus Conference on the use of Standardized Patients (Canadian Cancer Society, 1982) called for a significant increase in the use of simulations and clinical performance-based assessment and teaching. As a survey by Paula Stillman showed in the late 1980s, almost all medical schools had programs for teaching and assessing performance of students, most with clinical skills teaching and assessment centres and simulation patient programs. At medical schools and national levels alike, performance tests, and in particular OSCEs, replaced written examinations. In the 1980s, the OSCE passed a threshold whereby it was discursively one-and-the-same with "performance-based assessment". While Harden still talked about an OSCE that involved many tasks, ranging from knowledge assessment to use of models and to examination of real patients, others could no longer even imagine an OSCE that was not about interacting with a simulated patient. Sydney Smee, for example, commented that for her "when you say OSCE, I think patient encounters, performance-based issues -- why would you use an OSCE for anything else? ...If there is no interaction with a patient, it doesn't occur to me [that it is an OSCE]".

Gayle Gliva-McConvey summarized the history of the performance discourse the following way: Howard Barrows developed simulated patients with the goal of teaching and "duplicating reality", giving students a "hands-on experiential type of learning". Although he did create assessments, these always involved physician-observers and were fairly unstructured. Meanwhile, Paula Stillman was using real patients who had their own physical findings, to teach. She developed checklists for them to record what students did and didn't do. "Then all of a sudden they started colliding, because Paula started to use simulated patients to fill out checklists, and Howard was continuing to use simulated patients and saying 'the clinicians can do a lot of the clinical reasoning, but to document if the students asks or doesn't ask it...'

---

[9] The Report on the General Professional Education of Physicians (GPEP), was published in 1984 by the Associate of American Medical Colleges and called for a number of reforms in medical education, including a greater emphasis on performance based teaching and assessment. The GPEP report had a significant effect on reform in medical schools across North America, because its recommendations were incorporated into the accreditation standards for medical schools.

that is where they collided". She noted that when this work came together with Harden's multi-station examination, the OSCE was born.

As the performance discourse rose to dominance, there were signs of resistance. But the evidence suggests that the psychometric and production discourses that arose subsequently did not do so as resistance to the performance discourse per se. Rather, I will argue, these new discourses appropriated much of the language and methods of performance discourse and transformed them into a new set of imperatives and values. It would not be inaccurate to describe the psychometric and production discourses as "mutated" forms of the performance discourse. I have characterized the key arguments associated with these two discourses in the two chapters that follow, but I have not included them in my consideration of resistance to the performance discourse because I see them as modified forms of it. By contrast, I did discover several lines of argument directly opposed to the performance discourse, aiming not to change it into something else, but to critique its very nature.

5.41   The Split of Knowledge and Performance

Jean Ker, Director of Clinical Skills at Dundee spoke within a discourse of performance that is the legacy of her university. However, she spoke of a major objection to performance discourse and was one of very few at Dundee to question the root arguments of the discourse. As I have outlined, those who advanced the performance discourse argue that an excessive focus on competence-as-knowledge is misplaced and even dangerous for patients. According to this argument, doctors might be very knowledgeable in terms of facts, but if they are not able to demonstrate appropriate behaviours, they will not be competent. Miller's pyramid placed "shows" above "knows" in a deliberate move to value behaviour over knowledge. And while it might be argued that knowledge is necessary for appropriate performance, this is not usually the argument advanced for performance-based assessment. Rather, much of the literature and many of the key informants argue that the demonstration of skills is an end in itself.

Jean Ker questioned these assumptions. In her words, "[e]verybody says that we're trying to move away from knowledge to skills. But if you don't have the knowledge,

124

you can't really demonstrate the skill. What the OSCE assumes is that you have the knowledge already most of the time." She went on to argue that although she thinks that knowledge and skills have been falsely separated, she recognizes that there are important reasons for people to champion performance rather than knowledge. In her words, "[y]ou have to be very careful in terms of funding and how people perceive things, because knowledge seems to be a bad thing these days". She called performance discourse a "trend" and noted that "skills and attitudes are [considered] good". Studying "professionalism" is even more trendy she noted, while studying knowledge is outmoded and even rejected. When I asked her to speculate on why the study of knowledge might have fallen out of favour in place of skills, her hypothesis was that "Joe Public has access to all that knowledge, he can tell you the latest treatment of x,y and z. So how can I say 'I'm a professional and you're not'?" The answer, said Ker, was to shift the focus to the *application* of knowledge, a domain that could be claimed as an exclusive competence of professionals, certified through examinations designed to detect it presence through direct behavioural observation.

Another informant who told me that he was not very happy with the metaphor of Miller's pyramid was Danny Klass at the College of Physician and Surgeons of Ontario. He argued, "It's too reductionist for me. I've always had a problem with the fact that the peak of the triangle is the smallest piece, but it's really the biggest piece". Even more critically, Geoff Norman, editor of the journal *Advances in Health Sciences Education,* wrote a 2005 editorial arguing that "at this juncture, the Miller pyramid has done more harm than good" (Norman, 2005a). His reasoning was that "the subliminal message is that the ultimate assessment is performance assessment, and everything else is second best". Norman argued that there are two strong reasons to doubt the pre-eminence of performance. First, he argued, research on expertise shows that "you become an expert by knowing a great deal about a domain -- forget about skills". Second, he pointed out, "the correlation on knowledge tests and performance tests are embarrassingly high", suggesting that "performance and knowledge are not separate domains". He argued that "the Miller pyramid is now being used as a kind of statute; it's kind of like medieval monks ... all the performance assessment simulation freaks walk with this great pyramid in front of them". The result, he concluded, is that "you've got a knowledge assessment culture, and a performance assessment culture, and the two are shouting at each other. The boundaries are far more blurred than they're making it out to be". He concluded that "performance tests are an addition to knowledge tests, but are not a replacement for them because they are far too inefficient".

5.42 'Real' Patients versus Simulations

The second major resistance to the performance discourse as it has developed relates to its strong and perhaps now almost exclusive link with simulations. While the performance discourse included, in the beginning, advocacy for the active involvement of 'real' patients, this did not last long. As I have detailed above, Paula Stillman's work on patient instructors was taken up in a few locations, but remained marginal. While there are scattered examples of patients teaching (Bell, 2006) and gynaecological teaching associates are still active in some schools, the imperative to examine performance has taken on a remarkably similar form in most places. Performance testing involves standardized patients who are now routinely employed by medical schools portraying the role of patients for purposes of practice. There is rarely any interaction between standardized patients and real patients. More and more, standardized patients themselves have professionalized and taken on the characteristics and functions of the medical faculty. Many are themselves now faculty members.

Participants I interviewed were at a loss to explain this loss of the role of 'real' patients. Klass speculated that it might be tied to a shift in the performance discourse itself. He noted that a very early study in the 1950s argued that there were only two major factors active in oral examinations: "thinking about the problem" and "relational factors to the patient". He argued that for many years the second was forgotten and "medicine itself became very narcissistic and doctor-centric and they forgot about the patient in the equation. It all became like a cerebral puzzle for the doctor to figure out what was wrong with the patient, and the patient became like a bystander". The early introduction of patient educators and simulated patients, he maintained, went some way towards reintroducing the patient perspective. Others argued, however, that the shift of the patient instructors and SPs to more formalized roles as assessors and members of faculties of medicine have meant that this patient presence has been somewhat lost, or at least only indirectly represented. Some such as

Klass argue that "the power of standardized patients is that they bring something of the public into the assessment of physicians". But, many participants argued, while much simulation and performance-based teaching focuses on issues such as communication skill and doctor-patient relationships, in examinations settings there is often little or no time for feedback.

One of the students I interviewed said, "the one concern I have [with SPs and OSCEs] is that it becomes somewhat easier to fake things". This concern was expressed in a recent article by two sociologist who posited that too much emphasis on teaching and testing in simulated environments might result in the creation "simulation doctors" who act out a good relationship with their patients but have no authentic connection with them (Hanna & Fins, 2006). One student told me, "the only time that I feel like [I am] faking is when [I] try to be empathic. It is odd, I think, to express empathy to somebody when you know they don't really have the condition". Another student illustrated the degree to which OSCE examinations can become more about performance than about good medical care. This student said, "there is a huge anxiety component [to OSCEs]. I am not sure I will be taking beta-blockers, but we'll see. It's strongly encouraged by our program directors". Surprised that faculty would recommend that students take medications prior to an examination I pressed the issue. The student relied, "Yes, it is encouraged to make sure that at least we don't have palpitations and extreme sweating" when performing.

5.5   Summary

A performance discourse, emphasizing observation of behaviour rather than cognitive measures of human performance, rose to prominence in medical education in the 1960s. This led to the creation of new methods of teaching and assessment that focused on the performance of skills in real or simulated clinical settings. The rise of the performance discourse also led to new roles in the medical school for patient instructors and simulated patients. Dundee and McMaster Universities played central roles in the promotion of the performance discourse, when these institutions developed and exported, respectively, OSCEs and SPs. While the performance discourse is in wide use today, there is resistance to the privileging of skills over knowledge and the enshrinement of performance at the pinnacle of Miller's pyramid.

CHAPTER 6: CRONBACH'S ALPHA AND PSYCHOMETRIC DISCOURSE

6.0 Introduction

In proportion as it becomes definite and exact, this knowledge of educational products and educational purposes must become quantitative, take the form of measurement. Education is one form of human engineering and will profit by measurement of human nature and achievement as mechanical and electrical engineering have profited by using the foot-pound, calorie, volt and ampere (Thorndike, 1922, p. 1).

This chapter characterizes the nature of a discourse of psychometrics that began to have prominence in medical education in the 1980s and that is very much present today. Linked to psychology on one hand, and statistics, measurement and evaluation on the other, the rise of psychometric discourse created and advanced in tandem with the evolution of two new "subject positions": the arrival of educational psychometricians and transformation of simulated patients into "standardized patients". At the same time, these "discoursing subjects" promulgated and extended the psychometric discourse themselves. In this chapter I first characterize the key words and concepts associated with the psychometric discourse; explore the subject positions created by this discourse; examine the nature of institutions linked to psychometric discourse; and finally examine some of the implications of the dominance and resistance to this discourse.

.

6.1 The Nature of Psychometric Discourse

Psychometrics is a discipline linked to psychology and statistics that is based on translating human characteristics and behaviours into numbers for comparison purposes. One of the participants who trained in this tradition noted the importance of the origin of psychometrics in psychology. In his words, psychometrics was created so that psychologists "could capture in numbers psychological constructs that had no meaning outside a person's head". He continued, "things like IQ, like personality characteristics, all those sorts of things are human-created constructs that are abstractions designed to try to understand how people function". Put more bluntly, Canguilhem (1956/1980) argued that psychology "reduces its concept of man to that of a tool, and makes psychologists the instruments of an instrumentalism which is concerned only with setting people into place and setting them to work" (Rose, 1985, p.225). Given this orientation, the core task of a psychometrician is to construct and test predictive mathematical models and formulae through converting observable human behaviours into numerical form. A secondary, but important consideration within psychometrics is the degree to which the numbers generated "faithfully represent" the "construct". The ability to generate the same measurement with repeated attempts is called "reliability" and is a foundational concept in all psychometric analysis. So important is reliability that related concepts such as "validity" (whether the construct faithfully represents a 'real' phenomenon) are said not to exist in its absence. The goal of those working with a psychometric discourse is to maximize the reliability of data collected about human behaviours. Far from being simply a practice of mathematical calculation, maximizing reliability is at the heart of a powerful discourse that has far-reaching implications in how arguments are made, subject positions are created and institutions structured. Epistemologically, psychometrics is linked to traditions of science, positivism, experimental design and the search for "objectivity".

6.11   Cronbach's Alpha

Among psychometricians, the most widely-employed formula for the calculation of reliability is called Cronbach's alpha. The principles embodied in this formula provide a powerful representation of the discourse of psychometrics and for this reason I have called this chapter "Cronbach's alpha and the discourse of psychometrics".

Figure 4: Cronbach's Alpha

$$\alpha = \frac{N \cdot \bar{r}}{1 + (N-1) \cdot \bar{r}}$$

Santos and Reynaldo (1999) explains that Cronbach's alpha is an index of "reliability" associated with what is called the "variation" (or variability) accounted for by the "true score" of the "underlying construct". "Construct" is the hypothetical

129

phenomenon that a psychometrician aims to represent with a measurable number. The user's guide to the software package SPSS (Statistical Package for the Social Sciences, 2006), one of the most commonly employed programs for the analysis of data in medical research, contains a guide to the use of Cronbach's alpha. The formula is shown in Figure 4. According to the guide, "Cronbach's alpha measures how well a set of items (or variables) measures a single uni-dimensional latent construct. When data have a multidimensional structure, Cronbach's alpha will usually be low". The manual explains that Cronbach's alpha "is a coefficient of reliability (or consistency)". Embedded in the formula, "N" is equal to the number of items (e.g. multiple choice questions) and "r-bar" is the average inter-item correlation among the items. In other words, if students get a particular questions right, are they also likely to get other questions right? The formula calculates this relationship between the scores on each question, in relation to each other question, across the whole data set and produces an average. Thus "one can see from this formula that if you increase the number of items, you increase Cronbach's alpha". From this observation arises the imperative of psychometrics for "multiple samples" of human behaviour. Without multiple samples, observations cannot be shown to be psychometrically reliable.

The guide goes on to illustrate the second core feature of Cronbach's alpha: "If the average inter-item correlation is low, alpha will be low. As the average inter-item correlation increases, Cronbach's alpha increases as well. This makes sense intuitively in that if the inter-item correlations are high, then there is evidence that the items are measuring the same underlying construct. This is really what is meant when someone says they have obtained "high" or "good" reliability. They are referring to how well their items measure a single unidimensional latent construct. Thus, if you have multi-dimensional data, Cronbach's alpha will generally be low for all items". This characteristic of the calculation of reliability -- a need to identify "uni-dimensional constructs" -- has enormous implications as well. In particular, the units or "subjects" measured must be as homogeneous as possible in all dimensions except for the one "dependent variable" under study.

The number generated by Cronbach's alpha, the alpha coefficient, ranges in value from 0 to 1 and is used to describe the reliability of factors extracted from dichotomous (that is, test items with two possible answers) and/or multi-point formatted questionnaires or scales (such as rating scales where 1 = poor, 5 = excellent) (Santos & Reynaldo, 1999). In general, the higher the alpha, the more reliable the generated score is considered and therefore, according to the psychometric discourse, the more legitimate the instrument or test generating that score. Nunnaly (1978) has indicated 0.7 to be an acceptable reliability coefficient but in medical education, a figure of 0.8 is often cited.

It is important to relate the methods of psychometrics (such the calculation of Cronbach's alpha) with the epistemology that underlies this version of the positivist paradigm. The central goal underlying the effort to convert human behaviours and characteristics to numbers, at least in relation to assessment, is prediction. Using a predictive model, the scores obtained on an examination or other measurement should bear some relationship to scores or measure obtained at some future time. The hope is that by demonstrating the relationship of scores obtained at two intervals, that the numbers generated represent 'real' phenomena that also have a relationship. The challenge in this model is that the relation between human variables across time and place is always considered indirect, as it must first be transformed (in order to be measured) into numbers. Thus, psychometricians are particularly concerned with the process by which that transformation takes place and the degree to which the transformation is consistent (reliable) and free of distortion (error variance). The measures that capture the degree to which 'real world' phenomena are converted appropriately to numbers has been achieved, are themselves also numerical.

As with the performance discourse discussed in the previous chapter, the concept of validity is also important in psychometric discourse. Unlike its use in the former, with the links to authenticity and the 'reality' of clinical contexts, validity within the psychometric discourse is a numerical construct. Resting on a foundation of reliability established by statistical tests using Cronbach's alpha, psychometric validity is determined by further statistical comparisons to other data sets. For example, comparing OSCE scores to other tests of performance, such written tests, might be used to determine "concurrent validity". The correlations of scores on a medical school OSCE with those on a licensure OSCE might be used to establish "predictive validity". Finally, demonstrating that scores on an OSCE are higher for residents than medical students on the same OSCE might be used to demonstrate "construct validity". "Face validity" relates to the degree to which participants find an OSCE to be 'realistic' in its simulations but within the psychometric discourse, this is considered the weakest form of validity and is generally discounted as being of little use.

6.12   Key Words and Concepts

As I pointed out in Chapter 4, a whole new vocabulary emerged in the field of medical education in the 1980s. In fact, this was largely a vocabulary imported from the fields of measurement, experimental psychology and psychometrics. Largely the domain of psychometricians initially, this discourse was adopted by clinicians and educators already working in assessment and by the newly created "standardized patients". Table 5 below reviews the key terms and concepts associated with the discourse of psychometrics.

Table 5: Key Words, Concepts and Roles Related to Psychometric Discourse

Key words
Reliability, validity, generalizability, data, psychometrician, candidate, generalizability, item-banking, standard setting, cut-points, standardization
'Standardized patient' replaces all other terms for simulation 'Reliability and validity' appear in most articles related to assessment of any kind 'Generalizability' theory developed and entered medical education articles Students more often called 'candidates' or 'subjects'
Key concepts Exam quality, accountability and defensibility related to psychometric properties of tests Fewer references to teaching and feedback, more to testing
Key roles Psychometricians, PhD holders in psychology and measurement Some MDs and health professionals trained in measurement Rise of institutions with expertise in testing

6.121 SPs and Standardized Examination Conditions

As psychometric discourse gained prominence in medical education, the OSCE was viewed as one of the best tools for converting student performances into numerical scores. As I have emphasized, a key threshold in the shifting discourse was the adoption of the term "standardized patient" to replace "simulated patient" in about 1980. Wallace noted that the term "standardized" became "generally accepted" when the focus of medical education research "turned sharply toward research in clinical performance evaluation" (Wallace, 1997). I have already reviewed a good example of the adoption of this new discourse by Howard Barrows (1993). As noted in Chapter 5, Paula Stillman, who had written many articles in the 1970s about means of bringing performance into the classroom and who had created roles for non-physician health professionals and patients to teach, also shifted strongly to the psychometric discourse in the 1980s. She began to collaborate with rising figures in the psychometric world as illustrated by a paper she published with several measurement and evaluation specialists in 1986 entitled, "Assessing clinical skills of residents with standardized patients". In this paper, she completely adopted the new psychometric terminology, writing that, "Current techniques do not provide a reproducible, reliable, or valid basis for assessing clinical skills. The need for large-scale direct observation and standardized assessment procedures has precluded development of better techniques". The paper presented the results of a controlled experiment and concluded that "reproducible assessment of the clinical skills could be achieved in approximately one day of testing time using standardized patients" (Stillman et al., 1986, p. 762).

Stillman continued this theme in a 1987 paper called "Ensuring the Clinical Competence of Medical School Graduates through Standardized Patients", in which she once again wrote that:
There are substantial problems with the clinical training provided to medical students and with the assessment procedure used by medical schools to ensure that students have acquired the clinical skills necessary for graduate medical education. These skills are not evaluated carefully or systematically at any point in training or licensure. This article describes the use of standardized patients to help resolve some of these shortcomings (Stillman et al., 1986, p. 762).

Here again she made a strong break with her previous creative work in the classroom, now focussing on the "problems" of clinical assessment and the need to "ensure the competence of medical graduates" through rigorous, standardized, and *psychometrically sound* methods.

Marjorie Davis, introduced in Chapter 5 as the current Director of the Centre for Medical Education in Dundee, recalled that it was not easy to move to an "objective" system of examinations. First, medical faculty had to learn new concepts related to fairness in examinations. In adopting a model used for pathology specimens for live patients, she said, "we did a lot of convincing people to move from the status quo, which was the long case and the short case to this new method". She noted that this change required "evidence" and that the appearance of publications in the *British Medical Journal* and *The Lancet* showing "significant differences [in student scores] depending on which examiner they met in the exam" began to provide this evidence. The emergence of a psychometric argument that fairness was based on reliability, which itself required multiple observations, was one frequently advanced to support the move toward OSCEs in the late 1970s and early 1980s in Scotland and beyond.

When the discourse of psychometrics was new, and did not have much caché on its own, other arguments were marshalled to discredit standard practices such as the traditional oral exam, with its judgments of clinical competence left in the hands of one or two senior examiners. Davis, for example, provided the example of oral examiners coming back from lunch having drunk too much alcohol and failing students. Examples such as this were important in advancing the emerging discourse of psychometrics against a rather strongly held belief in "subjective" assessment methods such as "traditional" oral exams. Indeed, the use of the word "traditional" in association with oral examinations was a rhetorical device that created a sense that they were "outdated". Because it was not possible to convince physician faculty using arguments of reliability or measurement principles alone, fairness in examinations was raised repeatedly in the early days of psychometric discourse and conflated with standardized examination conditions.

Paul Preece, a surgeon and one of the first faculty members to be involved with the OSCE at Dundee, argued that the success of the OSCE was tied to the credibility of sampling and "looking objectively". He contrasted this (as is frequently done) with the "subjectivity" (and implied unfairness) of unstructured oral exams. He claimed that "[students] were frequently robbed at examinations" since examiners were often "prejudiced". In his view, the OSCE brought a degree of objectivity that overcame this arbitrariness. In his words, "[y]our person with preoccupations became a tiny part". Finally, he noted, this was accomplished because the "minute construction of checklists was [considered] the route to objectivity". Discredited in the 1970s, the oral examination was portrayed as an unwieldy and unfair enactment of power of professors over students.

6.122 Reliability, Checklists and Multiple Samples

Slowly, the concept of fairness was linked to particular psychometric properties of OSCEs. First among these was reliability, the key psychometric concept that is synonymous with "reproducibility" and "consistency". In an OSCE, reliability is the statistical measure of the degree to which performance in one scenario or with one set of ratings correlates with performance on other scenarios or sets of ratings. Although psychometricians would work towards the use of measures such as Cronbach's alpha to establish the reliability of large scale examinations, at first, the only examinations to be studied were the orals with only one or two interactions and one or two examiners. Initially therefore, the type of "reliability" most discussed was "inter-rater reliability". A number of studies were done to show that the scores of two examiners in traditional oral examinations were discrepant (e.g. McGuire, 1966) and by extension "subjective" and "unfair". The solution was "objectivity" and "standardization". The first was realized the by creation of checklists of behaviour elements that were evaluated for all student performances. The second was realized by using the same clinical material for all students. Where people were concerned, this meant standardizing the patients.

While the arguments of objectivity and standardization initially revolved around fairness to students, the psychometric discourse changed over time, as did the kinds of reliability that were measured. Very early on, people stopped using two examiners in OSCE stations and today it is virtually unheard of to have more than one person rating a performance. "Inter-rater reliability", the measure of fairness, was no longer taken

136

to be relevant since what was being measured was considered to be easily observable on scales with behavioural anchor points. The dominant measure became "inter-station reliability". Here, the important element was that the numbers generated by rating performances at multiple stations correlated with *each other*. The imperative was to demonstrate that the examination was testing a "homogeneous construct", that being competence in a particular skill. The use of this measurement of consistency (most often calculated as Cronbach's alpha) was much less often linked to fairness or the student experience, but rather it became associated with the "integrity of the examination" and its "psychometric acceptability". Evidence of high reliability was necessary for "standards of assessment" that were in-turn often required for defensibility. Defensibility would be necessary in the case that students appealed or launched a legal challenge against the examination (which is fairly common in medical schools when students fail).

Sean McAleer, the psychometrician in Dundee whose views were discussed earlier, provided a clear description of the arguments used to advance psychometric analysis and OSCEs. He gave three supporting arguments. The first was that "accountability was becoming a big word in the 1990s…[and] the exams had to show that anyone coming through the system was capable". Second was the argument that "litigation was just creeping in then". Third, he recalled, "the bad doctor syndrome was hitting the press". The trio of accountability, litigation and media attention, he emphasized, led colleges to feel they "had to do something and that something was to sort our exams out". McAleer told me that this "sorting out" meant moving from old-style examinations to newer ones that could ensure that "anybody coming through these exams is competent and capable". He noted that the words "objective" and "structured" were a big plus "for those who wanted to improve their exam in that context".

Geoff Norman, the psychometrician at McMaster University whose views were discussed earlier, argued that when publications on the new Scottish OSCE first appeared in medical journals, it was not taken up in North America. The psychometric discourse that would allow the OSCE to later flourish in North America had not yet risen to prominence and the British formulation of "objectivity" did not take hold. He told me, "I guess I was aware of the 1979 paper in the *British Medical Journal* (describing the OSCE) but that was those guys and we didn't like checklists and that sort of stuff, so nothing really happened". Much later, checklists would be so much part of the culture of assessment in North America that Norman himself would write an article criticizing the over-reliance on their use (Norman, 2005a). But in 1979 at least, the idea of a multi-station, checklist-based examination did not yet find resonance in North America. This is perhaps because of the way the Europeans were framing the idea of objectivity -- as a corrective for the vagaries of unpredictable examiners. Norman suggested that a claim to "objectivity" was not what ultimately made the OSCE successful in North America. He remarked that, "it was clearly the right solution for the wrong reasons. They thought it was going to work because it was objective, but it actually worked because it was multiple samples". In this comment, Norman illustrated a subtle but important shift in the discourse that was necessary to support the adoption of the OSCE in North America. While the Europeans had created arguments for a concept of objectivity linked to multiple *observers*, psychometricians in North America were more likely to speak about multiple *samples*. Although the Scottish OSCE indeed contained multiple stations and therefore multiple samples, the pure psychometric definition of a "sample" does not imply observation or even a clinical encounter. North America in the 1970s had no oral examination to improve, and therefore the new OSCE was better understood when it was seen through the lens of measurement that put a priority on "multiple data points". Observation is not necessary to the concept of sampling and thus, as far back as the 1970s, there were people proposing that this sampling of performance could be done just as well on a computer screen or even on a paper and pencil test using "Patient Management Problems". Thus, when the OSCE was adopted in North America, it was taken on as a means of sampling -- one which could be modified or even replaced with any other means that could be shown to sample equally effectively.

Dundee faculty today are not certain that they can appreciate the way in which the psychometric discourse has taken hold in America. Marjorie Davis noted that the shift in emphasis coincided with the rise of professional medical educators, both psychometricians and "professional" standardized patients. She also noted the role of large North American institutions for testing which, over time, have become the most important employers of these two groups. "The insistence on reproducibility and reliability" she said, "has tended to take the OSCE along the lines of the drive for reliability. I think a lot of what is happening is a drive for reliability fostered by the National Board of Medical Examiners". Ronald Harden also noted the new emphasis on psychometrics in North America. He thought that "there has been a big divergence and I think a big difference culturally in North America and the UK on the relevance or importance of psychometrics. That was why in the late '60s and early '70s what dominated the whole assessment in the States was the psychometrics. Because it was felt that reliability had to be the gold standard. If it wasn't reliable it was discarded".

Glenn Regehr, a psychometrician and researcher in Toronto introduced above, spoke about the power that had accrued to psychometricians by the mid 1980s, noting that they had acquired the power to decide what was legitimate and what was not in assessment of physician competence. He pointed out that "the Patient Management Problem [PMP] died because the psychometricians didn't let it through the door. It was a wonderful idea; it was exciting and it was incredibly innovative; but in the end it couldn't pass muster as a psychometric tool". With regard to the OSCE, he said, the "OSCE for good or bad has slipped past the gate. No one I know of anymore is saying 'wait a minute, does this thing have the minimum criteria to make us believe that the numbers being generated at the other end are legitimate?' There may be some tinkering, but basically it is [considered] legitimate".

6.2   Subject Positions Created by Psychometric Discourse

In this section I first describe the general nature of the subject positions of "psychometrician" and "standardized patient" and then I explore in detail the career trajectories of my informants. These profiles illustrate both how discourse is "permissive" and "constraining". That is, aligning oneself with a psychometric discourse allows one to do and say certain things. It also prevents, or at least makes it difficult, to say and do other things. While both psychometricians and standardized patients are subject positions made possible by the psychometric discourse, I will argue that they channel power and legitimacy in very different ways. The observation that most psychometricians are men, trained in androcentric disciplines is important, and that most standardized patients are women who are not. Being a psychometrician is associated with a fairly high degree of professional status while being a SPs means struggling to be accepted as a professional. These differences are illustrated most powerfully by participants who moved from one role to the other, as I will illustrate.

6.21   Psychometricians

6.211 Psychometricians versus Physician Educators

The arrival and rise of psychometricians was linked to the shift into medical education of theoretical and analytic strategies taken from the field of measurement and evaluation. Richard Reznick, a surgeon and creator of the national Medical Council of Canada OSCE, argued that the OSCE was the first place where generalizability theory was applied in medical education. He said that, "we did our first experiments using generalizability theory to understand the effect of taking the exam in English vs. French, the effect of the SPs, the effect of who the examiner was, the effect of doing the morning vs. the afternoon. There were several others and the only technical tool to sift through all of those was generalizability theory. And Jerry [Colliver], Arthur [Rothman] and Carlos [Berlovsky] understood Generalizability Theory and could do those statistics".

He added, "I would have taken courses in generalizability, and I did, but I would not have been able to, with confidence, run the generalizability analysis". Thus, in the opinion of physicians such as Reznick, psychometricians were essential to running a large OSCE, in particular in relation to "quality control" of examinations. Quantitative, psychometric analysis of OSCE led to the publication of many articles in education journals, he said, and helped further the field and the careers of the authors.

The rise to prominence of psychometricians created some tensions. One participant noted that there "were a lot of people who made their careers on the OSCE". Prior to the OSCE, most of the leaders in medical education had been physicians, and in most cases physicians without any particular specific training in education. A few had undertaken master's degrees in education, but very few had formal training in measurement, evaluation or statistics. Reznick recounted his first few meetings at the Medical Council of Canada where he had been asked to chair a committee to explore the feasibility and implementation of a national OSCE. He told me that a member of this committee said to him after the first meeting, "it was great that [you] kind of got things kick started, but now there [is] a need for a sort of serious educator". What followed was a struggle for control, but ultimately Reznick remained in place as committee chair with psychometricians as consultants. There he would go on to be the first to implement a national OSCE. "It was a question of ownership," concluded Reznick.

As Albert has described, the development of medical education has been characterized by struggles for control in many areas, perhaps most importantly about who has "legitimacy" to speak on behalf of the field (Albert, Hodges, Lingard & Regehr, 2006). The fact that a member of Reznick's committee challenged him as early as the first national OSCE meeting on the basis of his qualifications as a legitimate medical educator illustrates how important this issue already was by 1987. The struggle for legitimacy and control pulled between two poles: legitimacy based on closeness to clinical practice and patients (physician) vs. legitimacy based on knowledge of measurement theory and statistics (psychometrician). This tension was one that would play out throughout the psychometric era. When Reznick stepped down from the MCC, there was discussion about his replacement and a number of well-established psychometricians were considered, but another MD was chosen.

6.212 How Psychometric Discourse Legitimized Assessment and Vice-Versa

Jean Ker in Dundee noted that "with assessment comes power…and it's attractive to a lot of people to write about it". One participant told me that "there were a lot of people who made their careers on the OSCE. You can argue that Jerry [Colliver's] career was spearheaded by standardized patient-based exams, David Swanson's very much so. Susan Case -- she did a lot of work when she was working with David. John Norcini to a great extent particularly in the standard setting realm. Reid Williams, David Blackmore, Carlos Berlowski. I am probably missing several". All of the above mentioned individuals are psychometricians.

Ker noted that the rise of a psychometric focus in medical education meant that the literature became dominated by psychometric articles on assessment. For her, this had the effect of displacing other types of writing, such as "innovative ideas about learning and how we can promote learning in our students". She noted the tendency to publish articles on assessment with an emphasis on "fitness-to-practice issues" and "public accountability"; both are related to "the need to provide evidence". The discourse of psychometrics was more suited to providing evidence, and in particular quantitative experimentally-derived evidence, than discourse about new ideas in medical education.

One might wonder why clinical faculty accepted the growing presence of psychometricians. From whence came their willingness to confer on them so much power over what was legitimate in the assessment of the profession? I put this question to psychometrician Glenn Regehr, who explained that "[m]edicine came to numbers very late. But now they have a very positivist description of science that is almost always involving numbers and so do the people who have come to medical education. And in particular medical education research. For a long period of time the only people who were going to have credibility were people who were very facile with numbers".

6.213 The Fusion of Psychometrics and Simulation

Geoff Norman, whose views were introduced above, has been an education researcher and psychometrician at McMaster for over 30 years. He graduated with a doctorate in nuclear physics, but took his first position as the coordinator of the Standardized Patient Program. He recalled that he "was their first employee – like patient zero. One of the first actresses was my wife presenting as a tired housewife with depression and duodenal ulcer". It was not long before Norman began to bring his science background to the work of simulation. In his words, "I would arrange the bookings and currently we were developing research on clinical reasoning which would involve simulated patients". Elstein's research work on clinical reasoning in the United States (Anderson & Harris, 2003) influenced Norman's thinking and he followed Elstein's move of setting up a "clinical skills lab". Norman also set up reel-to-reel videotapes and ceiling microphones for observation and recording in the laboratory.

142

If Norman's first exposure to simulated patients came with the arrival of Howard Barrows at McMaster in 1971, Barrows' first exposure to psychometrics came from those studies of clinical reasoning skills that Norman was developing. The collaboration between the two arguably led to a significant change in the construction of the discourse of simulation. The initial funding for the research unit was from the Ministry of Health. At that time, the research was "basic" in that it focused on elucidating mechanisms of problem solving using a cognitive psychology framework. Norman recalled that "we videotaped them and went through the videos and every statement they uttered was turned into computer cards and we counted it. One encounter was 300 computer cards and I worked out all sorts of FORTRAN programs to analyze it". This work led to Norman earning a masters degree in medical education through Michigan State University in 1977. In reflecting on his career-long focus on research, Norman contrasted himself with Barrows and Stillman. He saw them as making their main contributions as "inventors" rather than as "scientists".

In the United States, Jerry Colliver was one of the first statisticians to work on OSCEs. The interest of psychometricians in OSCEs was a development that would, according to Gail Gliva-McConvey, lead to increased acceptance and legitimacy. According to Gliva-McConvey, "until they did the statistical analysis of this methodology, and the reliability and validity and all of the '-idities', most people were still considering [the OSCE] as an innovative teaching tool". She observed that it wasn't until the late 1980s that there was an "understanding that this is really a valid tool in assessing". The two elements that she credited with this shift in acceptance and legitimacy were statistical analysis and research. Neither statistical analysis nor research figured prominently in the discourse of performance. There were some publications by Harden, and Stillman and others, but this was very modest in comparison with the explosion of data-based papers that emerged as a result of the involvement of psychometricians. As Gliva-McConvey noted, "Jerry Colliver brought in more psychometric '-idities', the reliability, validity, etc. and that brought it more weight and credibility".

6.214 Psychometric Discourse and the Production of 'Truth'

Foucault has written about that way that specific discourses make some phenomena "sayable" or "visible" while rendering others illegitimate and invisible (Foucault, 1969/1972). An illustration of this effect is the way that psychometric discourse was brought to bear on the social equity issue of "bias" in medical education. Colliver was one of a group of researchers interested in searching for systematic biases in OSCE scores that might be associated with gender or culture. His group apparently took up this interest as a result of a concern in the late 1980s at Southern Illinois University that there was gender and racial bias in grading. A study published in 1995 compared the grades of women and men and of white and African American students in the three years prior to the university adopting a policy of anonymous grading and in the three years after. This paper made allusions to the fact that gender and race equity were highly charged issues for the university and that the conclusions carried a great deal of weight. The conclusion was that "[t]he results showed no effect of the anonymous test-grading policy, which suggests that there was no widespread gender or racial bias in the grading of freshman medical students before the change in institutional grading policy" (Dorsey & Colliver, 1995). Having used a psychometric approach to rule out discrimination in marking at the University, Colliver and colleagues turned to similar work on OSCEs. At a time when the National Board of Medical Examiners was exploring the use of an OSCE for national licensure, it would have been a significant problem to discover systematic discrimination in such an exam. Thus, based on a series of psychometric studies, psychometric researchers gave assurances that such was not the case.

Specifically, although previous studies had showed some effect of gender on grades, Furman and Colliver argued that in "previous studies assessing the effects of student gender, standardized-patient (SP) gender, and their interaction on multiple-station examinations of clinical competence, SP gender was confounded with cases, that is, male SPs were used for some cases and female SPs for others" (Furman, Colliver & Galofre, 1993). "Confounding variables" is a psychometric term for the situation in which one variable cannot be distinguished from each other because there is some relationship between them. Studies are designed to try to "control" for all variables that might "confound" the data. In a later study, therefore, they examined the scores of 166 students who saw the *same* simulated case. About half saw a male SP and half a female. Based on the absence of differences in the student scores on history taking, physical examination and communication skills, the researchers concluded that "the interaction between student gender and SP gender had no effect on the students' scores and ratings".

A larger study that followed examined the results of about 280 students taking OSCEs and their ratings on five scales. While the results listed report that on one of the scales (personal manner) "women students were rated slightly higher then men students" and that "there was a main effect of SP gender", they argued that "the effect was not consistent from rating scale to rating scale or from class to class". Therefore, they concluded that "differences in ratings given by men and women SPs should not be of psychometric concern, since the ratings of men and women examinees are necessarily affected alike". It is important to note this argument that although there *was* an effect of gender, it "should not be of *psychometric* concern" since the "ratings men SPs and women SPs gave were similar". In other words, there might be bias in the examination, but it would disappear in the psychometric analysis because it affected everybody (Colliver, Vu, Marcy, Travis & Robbs, 1993). Thus, a research paper that showed the existence of statistically significant effect of both the gender of students and of the gender of SPs concluded that "except for the women examinee's higher performance in personal manner, the men and women examinees generally performed equally well with respect to interpersonal and communication skills, and they performed equally well regardless of the gender of the SP" (Colliver et al, 1993, p.153).

In another of the series of papers published in 2001, Colliver and colleagues explained that this line of research was important because "ethnicity has been a continuing concern for the valid assessment of clinical performance with standardized patients (SPs). The concern is that examinee ethnicity and SP ethnicity might interact, such that examinees might score higher in encounters with SPs of the same ethnicity". The study showed that "White examinees scored on average 0.12 standard deviations above Black examinees in encounters with white SPs, and 0.11 standard deviations higher in encounters with black SPs". Remarkably, the point of the study was not to problematize the higher scores of whites than blacks, but to rule out the possibility

145

that this was a result an examiner effect. In other words, the authors were focusing on possible bias of examiners, but not of the examination process itself. The conclusion was that "[t]hese initial results are encouraging and should dispel some of the concern about ethnicity in SP assessment, at least about the operation of an examinee-by-SP-ethnicity interaction that would pose a serious threat to the validity of the examination scores" (Colliver, Swartz & Robbs, 2001).

This group of research studies was relatively modest in scope and numbers of participants and addressed issues of gender and culture in a limited way. All of the analysis rested of the scores obtained in a set of standardized rating scales used in OSCE-type examinations. This presumed that the ratings themselves were able to capture the constructs under study and that the cases examined would be ones in which issues of gender or race could be readily identified. Yet it is reasonable that cultural differences might be more likely to arise in a case of taking a sexual history than in taking a blood pressure. Few would argue that gender or cultural bias is always visible to the same degree in every situation. However, the tendency to generalize from a few cases studied to all situations and contexts is common in the psychometric approach because "main effects", the term for the psychometric result sought in studies such as these, are considered to be systematic and consistent constructs. That is, this research looked to see if there was something that might be called "gender" or "cultural bias" in simulated encounters. That is a different question than asking, in what situations, with what individuals and under what circumstances do we see something that could be called gender or cultural bias? It is also different than investigating the gendered and racialized nature of knowledge, as this topic is pursued by equity theorists.

My purpose in discussing these research papers is to illustrate the power of psychometrics as a discourse and its method of showing the "truth", even when that truth is extrapolated from a small number of observations collected in an experimental context. The work of Colliver and colleagues can be cited to show that "there is no discrimination in OSCEs" and has been very important in building the reputation of this new examination as an objective, unbiased scientific assessment measure.

6.22   Standardized Patients

6.221   The Renaming of Simulated Patients as Standardized Patients

As I have detailed above, between 1963, when Barrows first wrote about his
programmed patients, and the mid-1980s, when OSCEs were in ascendancy, there
was a multiplicity of terms used to describe a person who was playing the role of a
patient for the purposes of teaching or assessment. The terms "programmed patient",
"patient instructor", "surrogate patient", "professional patient", "teaching associate"
and "simulated patient" were all in common use (Wallace, 1997, p. 5). A wide range
of roles and functions are captured in these terms, including the prominent aspect of
the SP as a teacher. "Patient instructor" or "teaching associate" -- terms used by Paula
Stillman, labelled that the person was active in medical pedagogy and learning.
Others used the words "surrogate" and "simulated" to place emphasis on the idea that
the actor was somehow representative of a 'real' patient, and therefore acting in the
patient's place. The wide variety of names used prior to the 1980s reflected the
diversity of roles that were imagined for these new players in the medical classroom.

Again, as I have emphasized, all of that changed dramatically in the mid-1980s, when,
with astonishing completeness, these terms were swept away and replaced with the
term "standardized patient" (SP). Wallace recounted how this happened:
The expression 'standardized patient' was coined by Canadian psychometrician
Geoffrey Norman, who was looking for a designation that would capture one of the
technique's strongest features, the fact that the patient challenge to each student
remains the same. The term was adopted and generally accepted in the 1980s, when
the focus of medical education research using simulated patients turned sharply
toward research in clinical performance evaluation (Wallace, 1997, p. 6).

Howard Barrows also told me that it was Geoff Norman who "created the name of
standardized patient because it signal[led] the advantage of the technique". For the
first time, the studies required multiple presentation of the same case. For research
and in particular psychometric purposes, value was placed on eliminating variance in
the measure of performance attributable to the patient performance. Thus a premium
was placed on performances that were identical. This element of standardization was
new to Barrows and caused a major shift in the conceptualization of the goal of

147

simulated patient training. Barrows himself was ambivalent about this shift. On the one hand, he told me that he constantly goes back and forth between the terms "simulated" and "standardized". But he later noted that he always uses the word "simulated" in his writing when he refers to the phenomena that he created for teaching, assessment and feedback. On the other hand, he recognized that the word "standardized" confers more legitimacy. In his words, although one might be "uncomfortable with standardized because it sounds inflexible to change", he found that in the process of "trying to sell this to people" the use of the word standardized instead of simulated "advertised one of its advantages -- that unlike real patients, this patient is standardized for the particular exam you are using them for".

When I asked Norman about his being credited with the change in name to "standardized patients", he gave a different interpretation. He recalled the strong competition between Howard Barrows and Paula Stillman for ownership of their "inventions" and thought that the tension was unhelpful for advancing work in medical education. "Maybe it was me, I don't know, but at some point [I thought] we needed a neutral term that would not be in one camp or other. And that's where the term standardized patient comes from". It is interesting that Norman sees the term as "neutral". It may be that Barrows tried to own the term "programmed patient" and Stillman the term "patient educator" and that Norman did not try to own the term "standardized patient". Yet, as I have argued repeatedly, the shift in terminology clearly was linked to shifts in power. In disavowing a personal role in this change, Norman suggested how psychometric discourse can flow through an individual occupying a central subject position within that discourse. Norman, as a psychometrician, was and is a vehicle for the expression of the psychometric discourse. His presence is simultaneously made possible by a psychometric discourse (the discourse creates the position called psychometrician), and makes possible the psychometric discourse (the psychometrician creates the discourse of psychometrics).

As noted, after about 1985, all papers used the term "standardized patient". In a survey of all US and Canadian medical schools, Stillman, Regan, Philbin and Haley (1990) found that there was "widespread use of standardized patients throughout the curricula" in almost all medical schools. However, in reviewing the literature that emerged during this period, it was clear to me that references to the role of standardized patients as teacher or as surrogates for the perspective of real patients diminished, while those related to measurement, assessment, certification and licensure rose. The shrunken and circumscribed role of standardized patients, at least in the literature, defined SPs as a group of people working as standardized instruments of measurement; tools used for the uniform assessment of students. Barrows himself had changed his discourse and in 1993 stated, "The significance of the standardized-patient technique in assessment is that it can produce a valid clinical test item to assess performance that has many of the same advantages of the multiple-choice question. It is a standardized item, can be given in multiples, and can be scored in reliable and valid ways" (Barrows, 1993, p. 448).

6.222 Standardization and the Loss of the Artistry of Playing Roles

As I have pointed out, with the rise of psychometric discourse and analysis, the centrality of teaching and of representing patients' perspectives began to fade into the background. In some cases the human essence of the individuals doing the work did as well. While in the earlier period there was a tendency toward objectification of the "model" in the classroom, the individual characteristics of the women did have some presence. With the adoption of the idea of the standardized patient, individuality became a threat to standardization. Standardization itself was seen as necessary for consistency of material presented on tests or for research purposes, as measured by Cronbach's alpha, and thus a premium was placed on training a cohort of patients to give identical performances. Individual perspectives, characteristics or behaviours in the testing or research environments were construed as "noise" or "error".

In her interview, Robyn Tamblyn, one of the first standardized patients who later trained as a psychometrician, noted the result of this homogenization of patients, who could no longer present the rich nuances that characterize messy, complex and interesting problems of real patients. In the 1990s, Tamblyn was undertaking research in which she sent standardized patients into doctor's offices to determine what behaviours and actions the doctors displayed in everyday practice. This research aimed at documenting the clinical deficiencies of the doctors. Tamblyn's idea was to take advantage of the standardized patients being trained for the Medical Council of Canada examination that was launched in 1994. However, she recalled that "[w]hat we realized then is that those patients, in fact, had been trained in a very different way than what we would need for the patients we sent into practices. [The standardized patient] became almost untrainable. We couldn't use them because they were used for the OSCE". That is, they were not trained to act through a variety of contexts, as would be required in the competence research. They gave the same performance regardless of the scenario.

Sydney Smee, Manager of the Medical Council of Canada national OSCE, also noted the shift in performance of the standardized patients as training for examinations took on more prominence. "Most of the people I know in this business care about simulation, but Howard [Barrows] set a very high standard and I don't know if anybody else has ever matched it. In the old days it was an art form. OSCEs require standardization; you don't put the same effort into simulation". She went on to compare today's practice of training standardized patients for examinations with what she underwent as a simulated patient working with Howard Barrows. In her words, "[w]hen I was being trained by Robyn Tamblyn, Gayle [Gliva] and Howard [Barrows], in the old days, it was driven by the clinical findings, and the clinical presentation. And you layered the personality on top of that. I think the theatre arts people are trying to maintain a clinical realism, but it's a character in a story, you know".

This set of quotes is interesting from a discursive point of view. Smee argued that simulation is not the same as standardization and characterized the detailed training and simulation that Barrows, Gliva, Tamblyn and others practiced as an "art form" now only practiced by "theatre arts people". In other words, it is an art but not a science. Secondly, she placed it as a practice from the past with the modifier "in the old days". Much in the way that the use of the word "traditional" conveys a former or outdated practice, her wording suggests that that the field has *moved on*. Third, she noted that this art form is no longer linked to OSCEs and distanced herself from this discourse by othering those that still practice this art form, noting that they are "theatre people".

Although she has passed through many career changes during which she has been close to different discourses of assessment, Smee told me that she is closer now to the psychometric discourse. This was apparent when I asked her about the multiple names for her professional role. Like others, she credited the use of the term "simulated patient" to Howard Barrows and Steven Abrahamson, and the term "patient instructor" to Paula Stillman. She had been both. However she identified personally with the origin of the term "standardized patient". She observed that "there is a small cadre of us – a professional group developing its own jargon" and expressed preference for the term "standardized" because she believes that "you can have a patient with real findings who is standardized, and you can have a simulated patient that's standardized so it doesn't belong to any one person." This formulation is important. That the patient's problem doesn't belong to any *one* person places an emphasis on the generic nature of the symptom or presentation, and removes the role of individual personality or characteristics. Thus Smee articulated clearly the core element at the heart of the psychometric discourse: that individual characteristics are "variance" (sometimes called "statistical noise") in the data that interfere with consistent, reliable interpretation. There is an imperative for psychometricians to eliminate individual difference in the service of increasing reliability. It is here that North Americans and Europeans often part company. This "noise" that appears to many North American psychometricians as slated for elimination is the very thing that confers, for the other medical educators, "authenticity" in clinical simulation.

On the other side of this split, Jack Boulet, a psychometrician at the ECFMG (Education Commission on Foreign Medical Graduates, in the US), argued that the word standardized patient "should be scrubbed". In his view, the part that is standardized is the portrayal, not the individual argued that "you can't standardize people". Boulet prefers that they be called "consistent patients", or by the older terms "simulated patients". He added that "[i]t will take years to get [the term standardized patient] out of the literature". Thus Boulet argued for a return to what Barrows developed in 1964 -- a flexible actor who can shift with the interview and with the context. For now, however, the dominant term is "standardized" and I found little evidence of it shifting back.

William Burdick at the ECFMG also noted this split in the professional expectations of SPs. He argued that the "interpersonal piece" is still present "because SPs value it - - it is alive and well". But he noted that "there is a dichotomy in the development of

SPs in the formal testing arena and in the teaching environment". And while he said that this split is clearly evident at the level of national testing, he also felt that it was apparent at the medical school level, related to the relative dominance of a psychometric discourse. As he put it, "[h]ow much compulsiveness the schools have [about testing] is relevant in relation to the role of psychometricians in the schools".

6.223 Psychometric Discourse and Career Advancement

Informants told me about the importance of adopting psychometric models, or working with psychometricians to advance their careers. Devra Cohen, Director of the Clinical Skills Assessment Program at Mount Sinai hospital in Manhattan, said that without the guidance, teaching about psychometrics and mentorship she received from Jerry Colliver, her career could not have progressed. Sydney Smee, encouraged by Dale Dauphinee and David Blackmore (the Executive Director and Chief Psychometrician, respectively at the Medical Council of Canada) undertook her PhD in measurement and evaluation. Even Paula Stillman, who was speaking and publishing widely on her patient instructors in the 1980s told me that "people thought some of this research was pretty flaky". She had the impression that when she "worked with a really good psychometrician [and] had very good data", she was able to disseminate her work more widely and it gained credibility.

The move to an identity as "standardized patients" was presented as enhancing both the legitimacy and the availability of work for the women (and a few men) who worked in this job. Glenn Regehr noted that "if standardized patients had stayed forever a teaching tool, [SPs] would probably continue to be a backwater phenomenon. It probably would have gained momentum over time, but not nearly at the same speed". He argued that the link between the discourse of simulation and the discourse of psychometrics propelled both the legitimacy and the employability of SPs. In his words, "[o]nce you can say 'oh but you can turn them into numbers. And we can now create numbers with more reliability and validity than we could create numbers before', the credibility and perceived value of that technology suddenly jumps out". He noted, however, his awareness of the problems that this has created for individual SPs. "The individuals with whom I interact have spent a lot of time indicating distress over the extent to which the evaluation agenda has overridden the teaching agenda. The individuals I know would prefer to be spending their time teaching" rather than "evaluating". Regehr was only one of several informants who were aware that SPs value being artists and professionals, rather than tools for testing. But, like others, he noted that "evaluation is how they make their money".

It is important to point again to the difference between North America and the UK as evidence of the association of the two terms with different discourses. The shift to the term "standardized patients" never took place in Scotland, and Jean Ker explained that "[w]e call them simulated patients" because their main activity is portrayal of roles and giving feedback. She felt that SPs have a role in providing assessment, but only in areas of measuring communication skills and other aspects of the patient perspectives. She noted that "real" patients are often used and that the emphasis is on creating scenarios that have the appropriate content rather than strict standardization. For Ker and her colleagues at Dundee as noted in the previous chapter, the term "standardized patient" never really had enough resonance to replace "simulated patient".

The interaction of discourse and subject position is evident in the career of Robyn Tamblyn, who is one of the main figures involved in the dissemination of the OSCE across North America, along with Howard Barrows and Ronald Harden. Now a researcher at McGill University, she started her career as a simulated patient. Wallace recounted her story as follows:

Robyn Tamblyn had been one of the first simulated patients trained by Barrows at McMaster. Her introduction to the world of standardized patients came while she was working with him as part of a neurological patient care team. When one of Barrow's simulated patients became too pregnant to perform at a meeting of the Association of Neurological Professors, Barrows convinced Tamblyn, who had never heard about the technique before, to become an SP. According to Barrows: 'She became one of the best SPs I ever worked with and in a very short while became a trainer of SPs and set up the first organized SP program at Mac' (Wallace, 1997, p. 22).

In our interview, Tamblyn recalled her disillusionment with nursing and the allure of the work that was going on at McMaster. She highlighted in particular the research aspect that, for her, became a source of academic pleasure and also the route by which she became internationally known. Howard Barrows was her mentor in a time when there were not yet any standardized patient trainers or program managers. Rather than staying with the simulated patient world, *per se*, Tamblyn pursued a PhD and today she represents one of the few women who have been both standardized patients and educational psychometricians. By way of contrast, Jean Ker in Scotland admitted that she had never heard of a simulated patient in the UK being a faculty member, manager of an examination or researcher.

By the early 1980s, Robyn Tamblyn had already gained visibility in medical education for her work with Howard Barrows. In particular, they had co-authored a book on problem-based learning. When her husband was transferred to a military base in Winnipeg, Tamblyn appeared at the office of the Associate Dean, Danny Klass. At first taken aback by her ideas, Klass "found out who she was and who Barrows was" and offered her a job as Assistant Dean of Education. This was a new position created to develop methods of assessment. Not long after, Tamblyn reconnected with Barrows in his new role at Southern Illinois University and they created one of the first multi-site standardized patient-based assessments between the medical schools in Winnipeg and Springfield, Illinois.

Tamblyn was later a member of the committee that designed the national OSCE for the Medical Council of Canada. With regard to the latter role, Richard Reznick recalled that she contributed energy and innovation to the process. He noted that her specific contributions included use of alternate forms for equivalence of marking, institution of processes of setting standards for scores, design of experiments to look at equivalence of the English and French versions, and so on (Tamblyn, Klass, Snabel & Kopelow, 1990). Later Tamblyn pursued large scale studies using standardized patients as a means of investigating physician practices. She was one of the first to correlate clinical practices, including clinical errors, with results on OSCE licensure examinations (Tamblyn et al. 1998). She reported that "licensing examination scores are significant predictors of consultation, prescribing, and mammography screening rates in initial primary care practice".

Robyn Tamblyn, like Geoff Norman and others discovered that in the Canadian medical education context, promoting a psychometric research focus opened up many

154

opportunities. They have gone on to be recognized faculty members with a high profile in medical education. Although neither is a physician, both command a significant degree of authority. For them, the psychometric discourse has conferred a legitimacy that would probably have been hard to attain otherwise in the physician-dominated medical school environment.

6.3   Institutions and Psychometric Discourse

The rise of the psychometric discourse was prominent in several institutions, both university medical schools and larger testing organizations. Below, I have discussed one university and two testing organizations to illustrate the relationship of the emergence of this discourse to institutional growth. The University of Toronto, although not the only or even the most important centre for the development of psychometrics thinking, nevertheless was heavily represented in publications and presentation at conferences that had a psychometric orientation. The Education Commission for Foreign Medical Graduates (ECFMG) and the National Board of Medical Examiners (NBME), both in the United States, were among the most important large testing organizations in promulgating the psychometric discourse in performance-based assessment. As I will illustrate in the next chapter, these two organizations later merged and their nature changed significantly as they evolved towards promoting a more corporate discourse of production. However their origins were decidedly psychometric.

6.31   University of Toronto

Simulation arrived early in Toronto and a number of individuals who would significantly shape and propel both simulation and OSCEs were already working in Toronto in the early 1980s. Anja Robb, the current Director of the University of Toronto Standardized Patient Program, said she became involved by chance. She was visiting Dundee with her husband, an internist who was taking a course with Ronald Harden on OSCEs. Robb's husband described simulated patients to her and she was immediately fascinated by the idea. It was the simulation aspect and not the OSCE that held an attraction for her. Having a teaching certificate and an interest in acting and in medicine, she started in a minor part-time capacity and soon became involved

155

in setting up teaching programs using simulation, in particular with the Department of Family and Community Medicine at the University of Toronto. She became involved fulltime in the mid 1980s when she assumed leadership of the Medical Interview Skills Course. At this time, the simulation program at the University of Toronto was not dissimilar to what existed in Dundee and McMaster.

Things began to change, however, with the arrival of Arthur Rothman and Robert Cohen, two PhD-trained educators in the Departments of Medicine and Surgery respectively. Under their guidance, the University of Toronto became involved with OSCEs. The university did not have the budget to launch and study an OSCE using medical students, but Rothman and Cohen identified a need for the province of Ontario to screen internationally trained medical graduates for further study. The Ontario International Medical Graduate Program (OIMG) was the first to implement a large scale OSCE, and from that program, a large amount of research on OSCEs emerged for a specially-created unit called the CSAU (Clinical Skills Assessment Unit). Experiences at the OIMG were later drawn upon when the national Medical Council of Canada OSCE was developed.

Robb noted that, although her original interest was in teaching and improving medical student skills through feedback, the OSCE enterprise came to dominate after 1987. During the years 1983 to 1987 prior to her involvement with OSCEs, she was, in her words, "involved more in the educational part...and that's where I learned the value of feedback as part of the education process". This teaching perspective, familiar from my discussion of performance discourse, would later cause problems for Robb. There was little room for teaching or feedback within the large-scale OSCE that would become prominent at University of Toronto and in the OIMG program. In 1987, the University's emerging program in simulation was moved to the IMG offices. On this move, Robb commented that "the leadership in the Dean's corridor felt that this was a more appropriate place and it would become a centre for clinical testing. Since this particular type of clinical testing needed standardized patients, it might make sense to have them housed together". The merger of the testing role and teaching role for SPs was one that would cause conflict. A substantial proportion of the SP program never accepted the discourse of psychometrics that placed a greater emphasis on measurement, statistics and research than it did on teaching and feedback. Several

156

attempts to merge the SP program into the IMG testing unit would occur, including a recent one in 2006, however a merger has not occurred.

Robb explained that moving SPs to testing and OSCEs was a "big order of magnitude change". She noted that what Harden was doing in Dundee was "more formative in nature", and even though it was assessment, "it was an experiential thing". In Toronto, on the other hand, Robb noted that the "high stakes" involved in screening international graduates led to "a lot of OSCEology and OSCE-based research", processes that "got people thinking about things like reliability and validity and how to justify the marks at the other end". Robb initially liked this move to testing because it seemed more "scientific" and "even more important" or "more valuable" because it was scientific. She said that it "felt scientific" because "the outcome meant something that could be proved by numbers". This last phrase captured the essence of the psychometric discourse. That it was used by Robb, an individual with an interest in performance and education, illustrates the degree to which the psychometric discourse came to dominate over performance in North America.

Although the idea of an OSCE arrived in Toronto with several faculty members, including Ken Robb, the visit of American psychometrician Emil Petrusa also influenced the nature of the OSCE in Toronto. Anja Robb recalled that "[i]t was Dr. Petrusa who was invited to Toronto to address the authors of the original stations that were used in the inaugural [International Medical Graduate] exam. He gave a workshop on what an OSCE really was and talked about the elements of reliability and validity and concepts of checklists and how to prepare a blueprint". These core elements of psychometric analysis, once introduced to Toronto, set up the psychometric discourse that would characterize writing, speaking about and implementing OSCEs for decades in this location.

Meanwhile, Robb and other colleagues in Toronto would not find total comfort with this psychometric discourse. Eventually they began to articulate some negative aspects of the approach. Robb, like Tamblyn, noted that being an SP for teaching and being an SP for these new "reliable and valid" OSCEs represented "two completely different jobs". She said "we have people that can't do both... [and] we screen differently for one than we screen for the other". Her characterizations of the two

157

orientations illustrated the constraints placed on a person working within one discourse or the other. Those working in the teaching role, according to Robb, "need to be more intelligent; they need to have reached a place of personal development where they can rise above their own needs and put the students' needs first.... It requires a whole compendium of skills that are not needed when you are working in an OSCE".

Robb, like Jean Ker in Dundee, emphasized the central place of "reflection", "self-awareness" and "feedback" for those working within a discourse of performance. The addition of the psychometric discourse "changed all that" and marginalized many of these elements. Feedback was virtually excluded as a result of "security concerns". Further, student reflection on their performances was never part of the instruments of assessment or research used in OSCEs. Robb characterized the experience of being an SP within the psychometric discourse as "memorizing a script". Although she said that SPs in OSCEs "have to play the role authentically and seemingly spontaneously so that it's believable" they are always constrained by measurement aspects of the examination and have to "know their job in the station".

Looking back, Robb said, "I would like to see OSCEs used more for formative assessments as part of education. That's where I think their greatest value is. You get to observe, people get practice and the students get valuable feedback about performance that they're so hungry for". Robb, after many years, has returned strongly to the discourse of performance. However, she noted at the end of the interview that she faces yet another set of discussions about fusing of her program with the testing roles of the International Medical Graduate Program. This means that the creation of "formative" OSCEs is not a process that she has the time or the resources to promote.

6.32   The Rise of National Testing Organizations

Throughout the 20th century, national testing organizations have gained more and more prominence in North America and have worked with licensure organizations and professional colleges to implement mandatory qualification examinations. As I described in the previous chapter, oral examinations were eliminated after 1970, leaving only written examinations at all levels in the United States and for medical graduates in Canada. The UK continued with oral examinations, but as I described, was very concerned with their fairness. By the 1980s, testing organizations in all three countries were interested in re-establishing the centrality of performance-based assessments, but not in the style of the old oral examinations. Emerging work on OSCEs and simulated patients led to exploration of these methods for large scale examinations. However, in 1980, no one had ever attempted an OSCE for more than one or two medical school classes. Thus the 1980s and 1990s were characterized by an intense development effort and what some characterized as a "race" to implement the first large-scale OSCE.

Studies undertaken at the University of Toronto and in the Ontario IMG program were important. They were central in the base of research that was used in the 1990s to support an argument for the "superior psychometric properties" of OSCEs. Grand'Maison and colleagues were to achieve a first in launching a very large-scale OSCE for licensure of all family medicine graduates in Quebec, Canada (Grand'Maison, Brailovsky, Lescop & Rainsberry, 1997; Grand'Maison, Lescop, Rainsberry & Brailovsky, 1992). Positive psychometric results from this examination were published and formed the basis for the even larger Medical Council of Canada OSCE that became a requirement for licensure for all Canadian medical graduates in 1995. For the purposes of this chapter it is important to note the key role both the College of Family Physicians of Quebec (CFPQ) and the Medical Council of Canada (MCC) played in employing and advancing the psychometric discourse. Both employed significant psychometric arguments in the justification of their large-scale examinations and both published a series of articles containing detailed psychometric analyses that would be used to support the development of similar large OSCEs around the world.

The results of the CFPQ and the MCC OSCEs were not convincing for everyone. The National Board of Medical Examiners, which I shall discuss in a moment, noted that the reliability of these exams was barely attaining the threshold of 0.8 that they considered the minimum acceptable for a large licensure examination. This was one of the reasons that they would continue to experiment with the OSCE for almost a decade longer than the MCC before implementing a national performance-based

159

assessment. Further afield in the UK, the Royal College of General Practitioners (RCGP) were also considering an OSCE in the 1980s. Sean McAleer at Dundee was a consultant psychometrician for the College in the areas of standard setting, reliability and validity. He told me that unlike the Canadian colleges, The UK College "balked at the OSCE in terms of its authenticity" and found it "too structured". Said McAleer, choosing a fixed station length "just wasn't authentic – some [doctors] spend one minute, some spend 15; they didn't like that aspect of it". Instead of implementing an OSCE, the RCGP did a number of experiments aimed at enhancing the validity of the examination. One of these changed the format so that the doctor sat in an office and had 10 patients to see in two hours. He explained, "they could spend five minutes with one, 15 with another. We realized to have authenticity we also gave them a tray with mail. We gave them a number of telephone calls; we gave them prescription pads so we could look at how they prioritized". Thus, while in North America the OSCE was on a path that would lead to its eventual adoption for all medical graduates in Canada and the US, in the UK, uncertainties about the method and the lack of powerful national testing organizations prevented its use at a national testing level.

6.321   The Education Commission on Foreign Medical Graduates (ECFMG)

The US Education Commission on Foreign Medical Graduates (ECFMG) was established in 1956 to "evaluate the qualifications of international medical graduates entering graduate medical education in the United States" (ECFMG, 2006). Through a program of certification, the ECFMG is the body that assesses the "readiness of international medical graduates" to enter residency or fellowship programs in the United States. To do this, the ECFMG sets examinations which must be taken by international medical graduates wishing to enter the US medical education training system. The ECFMG rhetorically links its testing function with the quality of health care and safety of the public. Thus their mission says that the "ECFMG promotes quality health care for the public by certifying international medical graduates for entry into U.S. graduate medical education, and by participating in the evaluation and certification of other physicians and health care professionals. Further, they aim at "improving world health through excellence in medical education in the context of ECFMG's core values of collaboration, professionalism and accountability" (ECFMG, 2006).

After the Medical Council of Canada, the ECFMG was one of the first national testing organizations in any country of the world to implement a large-scale OSCE. It was the first in the United States. This effort resulted from the work of a relatively small number of individuals at first. The "pioneers of the ECFMG", according to those I interviewed at the ECFMG, were all linked to Miriam Freidman Ben-David, a psychometrician and medical educator who moved from the Medical College of Philadelphia where she was an Associate Dean; Ron Hamilton, another psychometrician who had worked as an accountant; and Amitai Ziv, an academic physician and expert in simulation with a background in the Israeli military. William Burdick, who worked with Friedman Ben-David when he was an emergency physician at the Medical College of Pennsylvania, took over her role at the ECFMG and recounted much of its early history for me.

This group developed what would become the ECFMG clinical skills assessment (CSA) for all internationally trained medical graduates who wished to access residency training in the United States. Later, it would become the model for the final clinical skills examination (CS) for all American medical graduates. Most importantly, the ECFMG became a major influence for the uptake of OSCEs in countries around the world. When asked to reflect on this expansion, members of the ECFMG commented on the important role of Miriam Friedman Ben-David. She had worked first with the ECFMG, and later went to Dundee and over 20 years undertook many workshops and consultations related to promoting OSCEs around the world. I was unable to interview Friedman Ben-David (she died in 2005) however her history is recounted in a special edition of the journal, *Medical Teacher* (Roma & Oriol, 2005).

The ECFMG has played a key role in worldwide collaboration and dissemination of OSCE technology. It has promoted the OSCE model for national assessment that had begun with the College of Family Physicians of Quebec and the Medical Council of Canada. Years of research and an increased emphasis on the assessment of communication skills with the addition of a written note[10] helped to bolster the image

---

[10] The ECFMG, (now NBME) multi-station examination is called the CS (Clinical Skills)

161

of the OSCE (it was never called an OSCE at the ECFMG). Development by the ECFMG paved the way for the OSCEs eventual adoption as the national licensure examination for all US medical graduates.

6.322 The Use of International Medical Graduates to Develop Examinations

Only through passing the ECFMG examinations could a foreign trained medical student hope to access American medical training or practice. During my interviews, it was a frequent observation that in North America there was a strong relationship between of the growth of the use of the OSCE and the perceived need to assess the competence of an increasing number of international trained medical graduates. Danny Klass articulated this relationship by commenting that "[m]ost every program has some special impetus. Why is it that the ECFMG got into [the OSCE] before the National Board? What were Arthur Rothman and Robert Cohen first doing in Toronto? What were we doing first in Manitoba before we did our SP exams for the students? We were all using SPs to assess foreign graduates".

Late in the 1980s, Paula Stillman also began to have an interest in assessing international medical graduates (IMGs). Her first paper was a small study assessing seven international graduates (Stillman et al., 1989). The focus for Stillman had clearly shifted from the medical classroom to a frame of state governance and regulation in work. She described this use of the OSCEs as one which would "provide an objective evaluation of an applicant's clinical competencies" to see if "the applicant's clinical skills were comparable to those of a medical student graduating from a school accredited by the Liaison Committee on Medical Education". Passing it would allow IMGs to eventually "apply for an unrestricted license to practice medicine" (Stillman et al., 1989, p. 454). Stillman expanded on this work in collaboration with the emerging ECFMG and her work would help pave the way to their national OSCE (Sutnick et al., 1993; 1994).

In Canada, Geoff Norman noted this "use" of the international trained graduate during the development of the MCC exam. Said Norman, "I looked at the data from one of

---

examination, and requires students to write a clinical note following each encounter with a standardized patient.

the first pilot OSCEs and I could drag it out of *Academic Medicine* for you. What you'll see is that it's reliable, but it was reliable because the foreign graduates were so different than the Canadians that I said to them 'basically you are using foreign graduate as cannon fodder to make your OSCE look good. We settled our differences, but at one point I was really angry because I thought that they were pushing something that really wasn't psychometrically defensible". Another informant I interviewed suggested that IMGs were used as "sentinel chickens" in early OSCE research, drawing a parallel to the birds that are sent down a mine shaft to make sure it is free of toxic gases before the miners themselves are allowed to enter.

6.323 The Elusive Goal of a Highly Reliable OSCE

Down the road from the ECFGM in Philadelphia is The National Board of Medical Examiners (NBME), the major medical testing organization in the United States with a long history of examination development and a strong tradition of psychometrics. Over decades, the NBME has developed and refined examinations with an emphasis on written tests and in particular, multiple choice question examinations (MCQ). They have published guidelines for the development of assessment tools as well as standards for the psychometric assessment of tests. A key priority has always been the goal of maximizing examination reliability and, as noted earlier, the NBME has been a strong proponent that medical assessments of all kinds should have a Cronbach's alpha of 0.8 in order to be acceptable. When tests of performance were considered by the NBME in the 1980s, an early challenge was to try to produce an examination that would have reliability in the range of what the NBME psychometricians considered acceptable for written tests. However, it proved exceedingly difficult to achieve this goal. As previously mentioned the NBME conducted pilot tests of their OSCE-like examination for over 10 years while organizations such as the Medical Council of Canada and the ECFMG went ahead and employed it despite their own reports of not achieving the coveted Cronbach's alpha of 0.8. One of the informants I interviewed in the US told me that this created a dilemma for the NBME. In the setting of the national exam, it has been heavily pushed in the direction of reliability; said my informant "this poor slob of an exam that only had a reliability of 0.7 sits next to a mega-MCQ reliability of 0.8 to 0.9. That makes the psychometricians pale".

163

In summary, the interest of national testing organizations such as the CFPQ, the MCC, the ECFMG and the NBME was crucial in the transformation of OSCEs from a medical school-based phenomenon to a much larger nationally-implemented testing system. Two main barriers would delay this evolution. In the UK, as has been outlined, the barrier was the model itself. Seen as useful for the assessment of skills at medical schools, it was not embraced as a final hurdle for national assessment. A more critical interpretation is that no emerging national organization in the UK found a way to use the OSCE to consolidate its power or influence in medical assessment at a national level. In North America, the combination of large national testing organizations and the presence of psychometricians in those organizations led to intense experimentation with OSCEs and their modification to serve psychometric and institutional purposes. For some time, however, these institutional goals were held up by the psychometricians who were not convinced that this new technology would meet their standards. Eventually these concerns would be overcome, but as I will describe in the next chapter, what made globalization of the technology possible was not psychometric discourse, but a new discourse that invoked accountability, quality and the medical student as "product". This new discourse proved to be power in propelling large scale OSCE-type examinations. It is unclear if national OSCEs have ever achieved the desired 0.8 reliability on a consistent basis, but while the psychometric discourse was in full force, all efforts were directed to this goal. As a result, OSCEs were rigorously modified to create maximal standardization and remove as much variability as possible. Unless an element of the examination contributed to its "discriminatory power", it was eliminated. The result was an examination that vaguely resembled the OSCE that Harden once gave to medical students. The regimented rotation, the strictly standardized test measures and the collection of massive amounts of data became a testament to dominance of the psychometric discourse.

6.4 Thresholds and Resistances

There was already evidence that the psychometric discourse was becoming dominant, at least in North America by the 1970s in the decision of the NBME to drop all forms of oral examinations because they "lacked psychometric of reliability". This was an extraordinary development, since it meant that the only examination that remained for the assessment of physicians in the United States for many years was a set of multiple choice tests. Reliability discourse was used to kill the oral examinations, but in the absence of a reliable method of performance-based assessment, none was implemented until the OSCE was taken up after the year 2000. One of the informants familiar with these developments at the National Board explained that "sharp-edged psychometricians" led an assessment movement that "became increasingly narrow". However, in his words, "recognizing that clinical orals were psychometrically suspect resulted not in their being improved, but in their being dropped". The result, according to this informant, was that "in the eighties, when things were probably at their worst, all we had were multiple choice exams driving student performance".

Other significant thresholds illustrating the dominance of the psychometric discourse were the shift to the term "standardized patient"; a steep rise in publications about OSCEs that contained psychometric analysis; the development of psychometric standards for examinations such as the Cronbach's alpha of 0.8; and finally, the publication of a paper in 1995 in which Canadians Rothman and Cohen argued that performance-based assessment had become so complex that the analysis of the psychometrics should be undertaken by a professional psychometrician.

As the literature review revealed, psychometric discourse had gained prominence in psychology decades before it made an appearance in medical education. But when it did, the transformation of medical education was profound. That transformation involved the same elements that Rose documented in his history of the rise of psychometrics in psychology. These elements were:
institutional sites; professional agencies; authorized texts; systems for organization and dissemination of research and discussion; ways for formulated arguments; relations between psychologists and their subjects; styles of psychological experimentation and adjudication; objects and domains appropriate for psychological judgement (Rose, 1985, p. 226).

As I described in Chapter 5, psychometric discourse gained greater prominence in North America than in the UK and in Dundee, the psychometric discourse did not hold much resonance. Cees van der Vleuten (2000a), a psychometrician at Maastricht in the Netherlands, has continued to call for a reduction in what he calls an

165

"obsession" with psychometric reliability. At the same time, one of the North American psychometricians noted that, "the measurement people with whom I interact in North America are almost all psychometricians. The measurement people, if you can use that word, [or] the evaluation people with whom I interact from non-North American environments are not psychometricians, they are inventors". Not surprisingly then, more resistance to the psychometric discourse surfaced during my interviews in the UK than in North America. However, I did find similar arguments made in Canada and the United States. Resistance took several forms and I have outlined these below.

6.41 Diversity versus Variance

A key area of resistance to psychometric discourse is associated with the conception of "variance". A statistical concept, variance represents the "uncertainty" in a set of data, or characteristics of the data that need to be "explained" or attributed psychometrically. Statisticians sometimes refer to variance as "noise". That is, this component of the data is conceptualized as reflecting the variations introduced into performance by variables such as time of day, fatigue, sex, ethno-racial origin, personality, etc. One informant noted that, "what the craft of psychometrics turns out to be is to get rid of variance, to get rid of unexplained variance". The implications are that "the easiest way to make a test reliable is to make the questions look similar".

In an OSCE requiring diverse individuals to perform, the implications of "making the questions look similar" concern Danette McKinley. McKinley is a research scientist and psychometrician working at the ECFMG. She is one of a very few African American women working as a psychometrician. Her preference is to study and understand the sources of "variance" in OSCE data. I interviewed her at her office at the ECFMG in Philadelphia. She began her career with an interest in reading and learning disabilities. Having obtained a PhD, her interest in measurement and evaluation led her to a job at the NBME where she worked for eight years on examinations. She said she has always been interested in the "people behind the numbers" and looked at how scoring related to test-taker characteristics. She broadened her scope with projects aimed at developing performance assessments for nurses' aides and acupuncturists. Later, when performance-based assessments were developed for large scale use in medicine, McKinley became involved with work to "make the clinical encounter more psychometrically reliable". Despite speaking within psychometric discourse most of the time, McKinley made a point of emphasizing the role of simulation for learning and performance improvement: "I always appreciated the value of the OSCE as a formative instrument" she noted.

In contrast to the work I discussed previously concluding that there are *no* effects of gender or race adding variability to OSCE assessment, McKinley told me that she just couldn't believe that there would be no effects of gender or race in doctor-patient interactions. Regarding gender, she said, "as a patient, I am more demanding of my physician than my husband would be. Women approach health care in a completely different way. Male MDs are more into checklist stuff and not the handling of patients". She told me that she believes that the increasing role of women in medical education is changing practice. In her words, "[i]f your committee has six women and two men, that has an effect on the key elements of the test". Similarly, in terms of race and culture, McKinley pointed to studies that show that African-Americans presenting to emergency departments get different treatment than Caucasians in the United States. She said it was hard to imagine that there would be no effect of race in examinations. The effect seems even more obvious to her in relation to international medical graduates. She said, "we bring in folks, but it is not their native culture. Non-western cultures are different. For example, a male with a female addressing an issue of sexual dysfunction, what does that mean to them? I am interested in the cultural issues". She noted that although the biomedical concept of disease itself is rarely attached to race, the way in which doctors ask questions and select treatments is.

Diana Tabak, Associate Director of the SP Program in Toronto provided an example. She told me "we were doing a complex pharmacy role. We had a Sri Lankan and a Mexican [SP]. When it came time to do the interview, the Sri Lankan could not look the professional in the eye. So it gave the impression that he was more depressed". Tabak argued that this would have been a terrific point of discussion for teaching, but that it was a serious problem for an examination. She pointed out that in "a standardized environment, it becomes a problem because he doesn't look the same as everybody else". One of the students I interviewed also recounted an experience in an OSCE that illustrates the problem of race and homogenization. He recalled that the stem [station instructions] said "this woman is complaining of a skin lesion". The station was apparently designed to elicit a history for melanoma and ask for risk factors. But, recalled the student, "the particular SP that I had was very dark skinned, and although melanoma happens in dark skinned people, it is rare. It took me eight or 10 minutes into the station before I realized what they were getting at. I came out and [in the second part of the station] there was a photo of the skin lesion. It was a typical melanoma lesion on a background of white skin!"

As part of her work at the ECFMG, McKinley is undertaking research to explore these issues further. She said she studies "concordant and discordant" relations, or the effect of having SP-examiners of the same or different race or gender compared with the student. She and her colleagues have found differences (van Zanten, Boulet & McKinley 2004). She told me that she found that women students received higher ratings overall, but that women examiners gave lower ratings. McKinley also found that concordance was important in terms of cultural background. She found that Asian SPs gave lower ratings, for example, when the candidate was Asian. She admitted that the research was imprecise because a category such as "Asian" subsumes many cultures. She expressed reluctance to draw too many conclusions from this preliminary research however she noted the importance of continuing to ask such questions.

McKinley noted as well her interest in the effects of examinations in shaping physician behaviours. Regarding international graduates, she said, "they probably have adapted themselves to get here and get through the system, but I wonder what happens when they take that back home. Does it give them a different approach in their home country?" With "global migration", she speculated that the shaping effects of examinations might be significant. When asked if examinations might instil any negative behaviour, or actually work against good clinical skills, she replied, "I suspect that is probably true. It's like a driving test -- they are doing their best so they can get through the exam". Devra Cohen, also in the US, told me that many international graduates take courses to learn the skills of passing OSCEs. A large private company called Kaplan runs an expensive preparatory course that, according to Cohen, serves to "acculturate [international medical graduates] to a more American approach to communication and culture".

On the examination production and training side, McKinley also has explored issues of gender and culture. For example, she noted that the ECFMG has faced a high attrition rate of SPs from non-white groups. To address this, she has tried to change the environment of training. While SPs "still see the typical young white woman who is training them", McKinley has made efforts to ensure that they meet SPs from diverse cultural backgrounds and that the training materials they encounter (such as videos) are also culturally diverse. She highlighted for me the importance of paying attention to the work environment and to being thoughtful about how non-white SPs experience it. For her, the examination cannot be valid if it does not reflect American society. She concluded "I think diversification of the SPs in terms of age, race, gender and experience really makes a difference". But one informant expressed pessimism that these issues are important to most administrators involved in testing. "Efficiency, money, numbers" make these things "problematic", she said. "Everything that is · problematic, you eliminate".

Statistical variability and its relationship to validity was a subject referred to by a number of informants. One said that gender, race and culture are sources of "unexplained variance that psychometricians can't understand". Another argued that within a psychometric discourse there is a belief that "if it's not reliable, you can't make a measure out of it", but that "if you work so hard to make it reliable you often end up with an increasingly meaningless test". A third informant said that the preference of some psychometricians is to "only measure those things that [one] can reliably measure and leave out the things that make a mess. You know, if you can't measure something, why bother with it?" I put this issue to one of the psychometricians I interviewed who said, "if the number that is generated from a particular measurement instrument is not reliable and valid, it's highly inappropriate to use that number for any purpose because it's measuring noise". By contrast, one of the SP informants argued that, "the binary checklist completely constrains the standardized patient, who then is no longer a patient", but rather is someone who has become "the adversary of the student", thinking "I'll give you the answer if you ask the right question in a standardized fashion".

Against the powerful backdrop of the psychometric discourse and the imperative to eliminate "unexplained variance", research such as the preliminary investigations of McKinley and her colleagues is rare. Several interviewees in Canada and the US told me that large testing organizations have become quite sensitive about the potential for legal challenges to their examinations. If sources of "unexplained variance" were to be shown to be discrimination on the basis of race or gender, for example, this would present an enormous problem for testing organizations. There is already a literature that shows this to be the case for testing in areas such as intelligence that I have reviewed (Bernstein, 1990; Gould, 1981). For now, testing organizations can cite the psychometric works of Colliver and others to 'prove' that the OSCE is free of such problems. However, as Sosnoski has written, "the more we move toward specialization, the more we move away from diversity. Exams normalize; difference is unexaminable" (Sosnoski, 1993, p. 325).

6.42   Authenticity versus Reliability and Validity

A second key area of resistance to the adoption of a psychometric discourse in relation to OSCEs revolves around the charge that it is "trivializing the task". Richard Reznick explained that, "the biggest rap against the OSCE was that it trivialized the medical task, that it was very cookie-cutter, and it rewarded a checklist mentality, and 'unrewarded' experience. And I always said, this is good for first and second and third year students [but] it's not great for senior doctors".

Reznick told me a story to illustrate this point. Early in the development of a national exam, at the Annual General Meeting of the Medical Council of Canada, Reznick created a scenario with a standardized patient for use at grand rounds. The SP role was to play a patient with a case of acute abdominal pain suggestive of appendicitis. Reznick invited the President of the Medical Council to be the physician. Checklists were handed out to all assembled, including many senior medical school deans. The President took the history and performed the physical examination, as he was accustomed to doing. He sat down on the patient's bed and said, according to Reznick, "well dear, I see you're not feeling well and your stomach is hurting right?" The SP said "yes" and without asking too many more questions, the President said

170

"you know", as he pressed on her right lower flank, "I think you have appendicitis and we'd better get you to the surgeon right away, and I am going to do that for you".

This put Reznick in an interesting situation, because the President of the Medical Council of Canada had clearly earned very few points on the OSCE checklist. Reznick recalled, "I said, well this is good because you can see that [the President] passed wonderfully and he failed miserably. And it's our job to disentangle these two. To some extent, the exam is not made for this doctor who's had 30 years of family practice, and knows the look of appendicitis and can make the right decision". It is not clear if the audience went on to discuss for whom the examination *was* appropriate or what would happen in the case that an experienced physician was required to take the examination (as in the case of IMGs), but the challenge to psychometric discourse is clear.

Jack Boulet argued that "the negative effects [of using OSCE examinations] are that examination-related performance is less meaningful". This quote touches on the threshold between the discourse of performance and of psychometrics. Whereas psychometrics began as an attempt to describe performance and to turn human performance into numerical form, critics are now arguing that the excessive application of psychometric models and processes has trivialized performance. That is, excessive standardization in the service of improving psychometric characteristics (e.g. raising Cronbach's alpha), it is charged, has resulted in the actual performances being less authentic, less meaningful and less 'real'. Danny Klass mused, "error is unaccountable variance -- I always thought the way to deal with it was to account for it and allow it to be built in. I always thought that it had to be there. I was a bit suspicious of the exams that were too reliable, because then I would have known that they removed all the truth from it". Similarly, Shuwirth and van der Vleuten have recently written the following: "We dismiss variance between observers as error because we start from the assumption that the universe is homogenous, where in fact the more logical conclusion would have been that the universe is more variant" (Shuwirth and van der Vleuten, 2006 p. 298).

As I have detailed above, Jean Ker at Dundee described how the performance discourse was modified by and ultimately became contested as a result of the rise of a

171

psychometric discourse. She argued that psychometric analysis has often distorted the performance merits of OSCEs. For example, she argued that in medical classes, "we are often teaching them 'this is what you'll get a mark for in the OSCE', rather than think about why I need to do that". She went on, "I would like to see the OSCE format used in a more innovative way that isn't so strapped in by reliability and validity data or prerogatives. I think the problem is as we've tried to get it more valid and more reliable statistically; we've actually come away from what we were really trying to do in the first place". In a final few words that illustrate her awareness that these words challenge a dominant psychometric discourse, she added, "…but maybe that's heresy".

As noted earlier, clinical educators refer to "face validity", a concept that one informant interpreted concisely as: "do a bunch of people look at it and feel like it looks right?" One of the reasons that the "authentic look and feel" of things has never found favour with psychometricians is that "face validity has lost all credibility within the psychometric community" according to one of the psychometrician informants, because "it is a judgement and not a numerically verifiable 'fact'". For the psychometrician, if a phenomenon is not numerically verifiable, it cannot be 'true'. Thus, concepts such as face validity, and the associated idea of 'judgement' hold little credibility within this discourse.

Glenn Regehr provided an example of this split by noting that a common OSCE checklist item is: "introduces self to patient". Because nearly everyone does it, he argued, the item has little discriminatory power. The psychometrician will say it shouldn't be on the test, whereas "the person who is worrying about authenticity ends up saying 'you must keep that item because that's a vital part of the evaluation of the interaction'". During the 1990s, papers began to appear that argued that an over-emphasis on reliability and validity were leading to problems with OSCE validity. Van der Vleuten, for example, was quoted by a number of participants as saying that the community of assessment experts was "worshiping at the shrine of reliability" to the detriment of student learning. Later he went further and called for the return of long case oral examinations and the replacement of large scale final examinations with frequent in-training assessment (van der Vleuten, 2000a). Glenn Regehr picked up on this theme. As he put it, "I have a pet theory that there is actually a divide

172

across the pond with regard to emphasis. I believe when van der Vleuten stands up and says we have been praying at the alter of reliability to the detriment of whatever it is to the detriment of, I believe he would probably end up feeling comfortable if I said, 'to the detriment of creativity and authenticity'". Referring to Harden and the discourse of performance he said, "Harden's emphasis is more on creating things that capture the richness of the phenomenon than on capturing a replicable number that represents the phenomenon".

Rose's (1985) writing helpfully illustrates the links between this discussion about the nature of test items and the agenda of institutions in which testing is embedded. He wrote, "as far as devices of assessment are concerned items enter or leave the tests on the grounds of their ability to differentiate according to the norms prescribed by the social institutions in question" (Rose, 1985, 230). In other words, the nature of tests and test items selected are a reflection of the goals of the institutions that create them. For example, in the UK Marjorie Davis noted that she and her colleagues do not believe that psychometrically-validated checklists are necessary for OSCEs and emphasized that at Dundee, where there is an orientation to the doctor-patient relationship, global ratings were emphasized from the beginning.[11] Similarly, in the US, Gerry Whelan said, "I think we are fooling ourselves to think that checklist items reflect the essential features of a case". Interestingly though, he went on to note that further discussions about the nature of measures in the US would be irrelevant moot now that the national OSCE has been institutionalized.

Sean McAleer highlighted for me that institutions are changing their priorities and argued that a movement away from OSCEs is starting, particularly at post-medical school training levels because of the need to "get back into attempting to assess real life situations". His view is that structured 360 degree evaluations[12] will replace most simulated assessments in the future. Similarly, Danny Klass argued that institutions are becoming aware that psychometric discourse has limitations, observing that,

---

[11] A checklist consists of specific behaviour items (for example "asks about chest pain") that are scored in a binary (yes, no) fashion. Global ratings consist of more general descriptions of behaviour (for example "treated the patient in an empathic way") and are scored on multi-point scales, which often have a range of behaviour descriptors.
[12] A 360 degree evaluation is an evaluation completed during a clinical training period, comprised of a synopsis of a number of evaluations given by different observers such as a range of different health professionals who have all worked with a student during the rotation.

173

"psychometrics really wants to be able to assess performance, but while psychometrics is great at assessing the *capacity* to perform, it's not very good at assessing performance".

In Toronto, Diana Tabak told me that there has been a movement away from more rigid psychometric thinking about OSCEs. She said, "when I started, you had to do lots of stations to give the right psychometric numbers, and then you could relax a little bit, and you could reduce the number of stations and still get valid, robust statistics. But it never made any sense to me from the very beginning, because I saw students who could play the game and others who couldn't and the whole thing never seemed fair".

One of the students I interviewed recounted a story that illustrated how the numbers generated by OSCEs could become more important than the actual experience. The student recalled that there were "three standardized patients doing the same case. I am sure they did not give the same story in the end so the students didn't have the same flavour of the patient". These differences, the student observed, would have been interesting to explore to understand the variability in the presentation of cases. However, according to the student, the course director said "the marks are same, the average is the same" and therefore the presentations "must have been the same".

Finally, Ronald Harden noted that even the core idea that OSCEs are "objective" is not necessarily always the case. He told me that he likes to remind people that it could just as well be called a "POSCE"; that is a "Potentially Objective Structured Clinical Examination". There is nothing magic in its makeup that guarantees objectivity, he emphasized. He warned that "when looking at reliability it really depends as much on the group delivering it as the technique itself". Harden went on to echo the work of European psychometrician Cees van der Vleuten in saying that, "there's too much emphasis on reliability and quoting of reliability of techniques of assessment". He cited the key area of communication skills, commenting that "[i]n the very early years it was obvious, and you didn't really need psychometrics to tell you that if you want to assess someone communicating with a score sheet or global ratings or whatever, you've actually got to have a station where you watch them communicating. If you want to measure a reflex in a leg, [or] examine an abdomen, you've actually got to

174

watch them. There is no argument against that". And so the discourse of performance reasserts itself. Regehr concluded that in "the evolution of the technology into something which is numerically reliable and valid, you have managed to remove that thing which we started with in the first place. In essence, the world is a messy place; therefore measurement instruments that have any authenticity must be messy. Any effort to clean up the instrument for the purposes of increasing reliability and validity by definition is going to affect authenticity detrimentally".

6.5   Summary

A psychometric discourse became prominent in medical education in the 1980s and is in wide-spread use today. Emphasizing statistics and measurement the psychometric discourse created opportunities for educational psychometricians and led to the transformation of simulated patients into standardized patients. The discourse was also taken up and promoted by some medical schools, such as the University of Toronto, and by national testing organizations such as the Medical Council of Canada and the National Board of Medical Examiners. Psychometric discourse led to the standardization of all facets of OSCEs and to the removal of elements of "variance" that reduced statistical "reliability". Negative effects of an overemphasis on psychometric discourse include the disappearance of feedback, the de-emphasis of teaching, the homogenization of examination content and role presentation and the deskilling of standardized patients who work primarily in examinations. These have led to resistance including calls to de-emphasize the psychometric discourse. At the same time, the use of psychometric discourse is associated with greater power for institutions and with career advancement for physicians, educators and standardized patients who take it up.

CHAPTER 7: TAYLORISM AND PRODUCTION DISCOURSE

7.0   Introduction

This chapter characterizes the discourse of production that began to have prominence
in medical education generally, and testing particularly, in the 1990s. It is very much
a dominant discourse today, although more prominent in some institutions and
geographic locations than others. Production discourse is imbued with language and
concepts borrowed from manufacturing and industry. The rise of the production
discourse created and advanced in tandem with the creation of new "subject
positions" such as the testing organization administrator and the standardized patient
trainer. In this chapter, I characterize the key words and concepts associated with
production discourse; explore the subject positions created by this discourse; examine
the nature of institutions linked to the production discourse; and finally examine some
of the resistance to this discourse.

7.1   The nature of production discourse

7.11   Taylorism

When I characterized the discourses of performance and psychometrics, the symbols
and metaphors of Miller's Pyramid and Cronbach's alpha, respectively, emerged from
the literature and interviews as potent symbols of these discourses. No similar symbol
or metaphor was used consistently in the literature or by participants using production
discourse. Nevertheless, the key words and concepts that I encountered over and over
strongly suggested a metaphor -- that of Taylorism.

Frederick Taylor wrote *The Principles of Scientific Management* in 1911, and the
discourse that would become known as Taylorism was widely taken up in industry
and manufacturing. In his book *Management for Productivity*, Schermerhorn (1993)
summarized some of the key elements of Taylorism. These include:

1. Developing a "science" for every job, including rules of motion and
   standardized work procedure;

2. Carefully selecting workers with the right abilities for the job;

3. Carefully training workers to do the job, and giving them proper incentives to
   cooperate with the "job science"; and

4. Supporting workers by planning their work and the way as they go about their jobs.

In his book, Taylor stated that "[i]t is no single element, but rather this whole combination, that constitutes "scientific management". He emphasized goals of "science, not rule of thumb", "cooperation, not individualism", "maximum output, in place of restricted output" and "the development of each man to his greatest efficiency and prosperity" (Taylor, 1911, p. 62).

Taylorism introduced standardization of the work environment, the tasks of work and of the workers themselves, with an overall goal of increasing efficiency in the service of productivity. Becker and Steele (1995) have noted that Taylorism became a significant part of many kinds of organizations after the beginning of the twentieth century, and that it has been continuously refined and reinforced by major American corporations for the last 75 years. Kwolek-Folland (1994) showed how the uptake of these principles changed the organizational aspects of the workplace. In his words, "[t]he corporate order, with its assembly-line techniques, job differentiation, and increased organizational size, demanded a different type of office space and a more regulated and regimented flow of time". Thus many of the twentieth century changes to the workplace and to the nature of work itself can be traced back to Taylor and his "principles of scientific management". These ideas are readily identifiable in the production discourse related to OSCEs, including the writing on development of specialized testing organizations, the compartmentalization of tasks and workspaces, the creation of specialized divisions of labour, and a focus on the "product" of labour. Coupled with the prominent discourses of efficiency and productivity, Taylorism serves as an apt metaphor for the discourse of production in medical education.

Like the other two discourses, the production discourse contains within it a concept of "validity". However, the discourse of production involves a different use of the term validity than within the performance discourse (to represent the authenticity of simulation of clinical contexts), or the statistical tests that establish validity within the psychometric discourse. Validity is used by those within a discourse of production to mean the degree to which the test produces a high quality, standardized product. In Taylor's model, quality is assured through standardization of processes, surveillance of compliance with standard methods, checks of processes and outcomes, employee training and management structures that detect problems in production and extensive documentation.

As many scholars have noted, it is not just factories and industries that adopted production discourse in the twentieth century. Magnusson has highlighted the central role that universities play in producing theories and methodologies "that serve the growing need to 'rationally' manage the public and private sectors" (Magnusson, 2000, p. 111). Muzzin described the effects of the adoption by universities of discourses related to economic productivity in the form of academic capitalism. Four features of this discourse can also be seen in the rise of large-scale OSCEs. These are: 1. more direct research funding, hiring and agendas related to corporations; 2. a change in the nature of labour to incorporate a "logic of accounting"; 3. massive new investment into architecture and capital funding; and 4. an effect of corporate steering on curricula (Muzzin, 2005, p. 155).

7.12   Key Words and Concepts Associated with Production Discourse

By the late 1990s in North America, much of the attention, literature and development money that was being invested in OSCEs was associated with the interests of large testing organizations. The nature of what constituted an OSCE had shifted. Below (in Table 6) is a list of some of the key words that became common in writing about OSCEs in the 1990s as compared to earlier periods. These words were also used by participants speaking within performance discourse.

178

Table 6: Key Words, Concepts and Roles Related to Production Discourse

Key words

standards, competence, licensure, certification, efficiency, end-product, cost, cost analysis, investment, accountability, unannounced standardized patient, foreign medical graduate, international, global standards, international medical graduates, screening, language proficiency, rationale use, standard setting, expense

Key concepts

Development of testing institutions

Professionalization of standardized patients

Mass testing at national level

Key roles

Senior managers of testing organizations, scientists and administrators with large data banks

SPs and OSCE technology developed by licensure and certification organizations

Emergence of use of performance-assessment to monitoring doctors practices billing with links to government and health care organizations

SPs as lower paid labour to run large scale testing operations

A feature of production discourse is the prominence of words and ideas that are used in business, factories and mass production. Jean Ker, a medical educator from Dundee, noted that when she took a Harvard medical education leadership course in the late 1990s, the language and metaphors of business were used to discuss medical education. Ker recalled being taught that "production, at the end of the day, should have the same standards [as business].... What's important is the quality of the product that you produce. In medicine, we produce a variable standard of product". Sean McAleer, also at Dundee, in the spirit of the factory metaphor, called the OSCE "a great machine".

Much of the new terminology was imported from the field of management. This was illustrated in the thesis produced by Clark (2000) at the University of Dundee. This work was an analysis of the "organisational management structures related to the delivery of the OSCE" (Clark, 2000, p. 1). Terminology such as "logistics and line management process", the "chain of command" and "retrievable data storage systems" are found throughout the work. Clark used a quote from a management text that positioned management and production as primary to performance. He said that "a poor organization structure makes good performance impossible" (Mullins, 1999, p. 521, cited in Clark, 2000). Recommendations from his thesis included implementation of a timetable for planning operations; a "tighter command and control framework" in medical education; new positions such as an "assessment officer"; and the creation of a "clearer hierarchy".

Production discourse also derives from economics. Economic terms are commonly used to discuss large-scale national OSCEs, and they are also found more generally in the literature and other discourse around medical school-based assessment. For example, Anja Robb described the development of simulation in Toronto as driven by "social and economic factors", including the scarcity of funding for hospitals that resulted in a faster turn-over of patients. Specifically, with "fewer and fewer patients who were well enough to actually be used as teaching fodder", she suggested, simulation became an important alternative. Robb linked this shift with ethics; because, as she reasoned, "it's not ethical to expect people who are that ill to be part of the educational enterprise.... I don't think [they] have the capacity to give consent". In her words, the shift to simulations meant that "education could happen more effectively and efficiently because things could be planned in advance". A more cynical observation would be that simulation permitted "just-in-time education".

Similarly using economic language, Gayle Gliva-McConvey argued that in using an OSCE for large scale testing, the first consideration is "cost"; she thought such consideration were more important than "is it going to test what you want to test?" The primacy of cost and economic considerations makes the production discourse quite different from performance or psychometric discourses. The three discourses co-exist, but it is easy to pick out production discourse because of language that harkens back to early standardization of industrial production. Articles discussing cost and human resource implications of the OSCE appeared for the first time in the 1990s (Poenaru, Morales, Richard & O'Conner, 1997; Carpenter, 1995; Cusimano, Cohen, Tucker, Murnaghan, Kodama & Reznick, 1994; Reznick et al., 1993).

The links between production discourse and profit was often explicit in my interviews. Jack Boulet at the Education Commission on Foreign Medical Graduates said, "look at the companies! There are scoring systems companies, video system companies, simulation companies -- all are traceable back to clinical skills assessment. The original software company that helped us develop our programs now sells it to all the medical schools in America." William Burdick, also at the ECFMG, noted that the US national examination is based on a very complicated model that is unlike what has been created in most other countries. When I asked him why this should be, he suggested that it was related to amount of money needed and, in particular, the massive computer systems required to keep the examination functioning.

The corporate world also supplied production discourse with the concept of "intellectual property". As the original inventors of simulation and testing methods moved onto the international stage, they began to invoke concepts of "ownership". For example, there was a competition between Howard Barrows and Paula Stillman over recognition of their individual methods of simulation. This was reported by several participants. One recalled that "the two of them were inventors, staring down the other and talking patent infringement". Several other interviewees spoke about Ronald Harden's desire to promulgate the name OSCE, and Harden himself spoke of

181

others wanting to create and own differently-named examinations that had the same basic features. Glenn Regehr noted that he had encouraged a young surgeon developing a new multi-station examination not to call it an OSCE. The name finally chosen was the OSATS (Objective Structured Assessment of Technical Skills). Regehr explained, "you can blame me for the proliferation of new language because I said, 'if you call it a surgical skills OSCE you will not be able to make claim to invention as much as if you call it something new'". The reason for claiming a new name, according to Regehr, was that the surgeon was "evolving a new technology". Thus he argued that it would be "valuable for her to draw a distinction". Regehr told me that Professor Alfred Cushieri (who was the Head of the Department of Surgery at the time that the first OSCE was created), on seeing a presentation of the OSATS remarked "that's just an OSCE". Regehr said he agreed, "Yes, that's what it is". This is an example of how language is used to construct perceptions of difference, of affiliation, of invention and of ownership. Even when it can be readily admitted that the old term might apply just as well, a new term is invented in the service of promotion, branding and identity; these are all key concepts in the discourse of production.

There are limits to the prominence of production discourse. For Barrows, Tamblyn, Harden and other "inventors", I observed that the talk of invention and ownership remained at the *individual* level, and was connected to ideas of intellectual property and academic credit. Such claims and competitions were part of their lives as faculty members and I found little evidence that any of the inventors actually patented or copyrighted their inventions when the OSCE moved from the medical school environments to the international stage. Also while they earned money for talks and consulting, none created a company to sell their "product" and their work was published in freely-accessible journals. Further, all continued to move through a series of inventions, giving the impression that it was invention itself as much as ownership that motivated them. Periodically, psychometricians also spoke of control and ownership of data, but I found no example of a psychometricians starting a company or patenting an invention at an individual level.

As OSCEs moved beyond academia, and in particular large testing organizations, the discourse of production became dominant. Here I encountered discussions of "owning" the OSCE itself, or more specifically, particular "brands" of OSCEs. An association was also made between a certain type of OSCE and a person, program or institution. For example, the Clinical Skills Assessment (CSA) of the ECFMG/NBME is a registered trademark and the examination materials (checklists, scoring rubrics) have been copyrighted.

It is useful to compare the production discourse with the performance and psychometric discourses discussed in the last two chapters. Although the discourses of performance and production are not mutually exclusive, in medicine they have grown rather distinct. First and foremost, the production discourse excludes many elements that are central to the performance discourse. Elements of artistry, creativity, flexibility, control of scenarios by physician teachers and simulated patients and the iterative loop from assessment back to learning are all absent from the production discourse. Those using a discourse of production even emphasize the distinct role of assessment and its distance from teaching. Sydney Smee, Manager of the Medical Council of Canada national OSCE, for example, noted that when individual medical schools become involved with overseeing the Medical Council of Canada examinations, the requirements of examination production leaves little room for the creativity and flexibility that characterizes simulation for teaching. Large testing organizations do not provide significant feedback to students, nor do they see it as their role to do so. A student participant reported having experienced more than 12 OSCEs in her training and not one instance of simulation for the purpose of learning or feedback.

One might ask whether the production discourse really displaced the psychometric discourse. There is no question that large OSCEs continue to have a strong psychometric aspect. It is telling, however, that many of the original academic psychometricians no longer involve themselves with OSCEs. Glenn Regehr noted that the original attraction was "trying to advance science through psychometrics and advance the science of psychometrics". Noting the change in opportunities for psychometricians with the move to a discourse of production, he said, "I think the OSCE is going to be [of less] interest for them". Rather than building a career on OSCE research by getting grants and publishing papers, today's psychometricians work, as one informant put it, "in the basement at the National Boards" processing large amounts of examinations data. The purpose of data analysis is quality control, not research. One informant at an academic institution called the incumbents of these positions "psychometric technicians" and characterized them as jobs that could be done by "anybody with an SPSS package [who] can run an alpha co-efficient".

Several informants told me that the moment for intensive research on OSCEs had passed and that not many theoretical questions were still being posed. One psychometrician drew an analogy to the shift in publishing on multiple-choice questions, noting that papers on MCQs today focus on pragmatic issues of implementation, and perhaps quality control rather than challenging theoretical questions. This echoed the concern of Rowntree (1987) that I cited in Chapter 4 in which he noted that almost all literature on assessment methods is about technical refinements of tools. One informant summed up the situation when he remarked that "nobody is questioning … the OSCE. Now they're just using it. The tool is no longer the object of study. The tool is the medium by which studies occur". Another emphasized that large testing organizations such as the National Board are reluctant to publish for fear of the legal ramifications. Several participants noted that psychometricians, whose names once appeared on a flood of OSCE research papers, have moved on to other interests. In particular, there are no papers that critique the use of OSCEs. One informant commented that he was "not aware of anybody who's saying 'stop'". He ventured, "I don't think right now would be the right time to stay, 'stop, don't'. That's like putting your hand up in front of a flood".

7.2   Subject Positions Created by Production Discourse

Taylorism and the discourse of production are linked with differentiation and specialization of labour, hierarchical structures and an imperative for improving and monitoring the skills and performance of employees. Arguably the rise of production discourse gave new prominence to the "management" functions of individuals already working on OSCEs and assessment. As I have described above, psychometricians may have become technicians in the "data-management departments" of testing organizations, or left the field of OSCE assessment altogether. Large scale production also created new roles with administrative and management responsibilities. The need for managers to run large-scale testing operations led people from diverse backgrounds, including some clinicians, standardized patients and psychometricians, to reconfigure themselves as administrators, managers and in a few cases, CEOs. The arrangements for simulation continued, but became embedded in a hierarchical management structure. The role of Standardized Patient Trainer became more formalized. Not all standardized patients would become trainers, and some trainers were never actually standardized patients. Increasingly, trainers took on roles in human resource management, finance and other administrative aspects of production. Finally, not only did the rising discourse of production create jobs for people to become managers, administrators and standardized patient trainers in testing organizations, these individuals themselves promulgated and extended the discourse of production, adopting a language characterized by the key words and concepts linked to Taylorism.

7.21 Management

7.211 Pushing Through the Road Blocks to Production at the Medical Council of Canada

The Medical Council of Canada was the first national organization to develop an OSCE (although this occurred several years after the first large scale OSCE was launched in Quebec for all graduates of family medicine training). As I discussed in detail above, interviewees commented on the greater rapidity in the implementation of this examination in Canada (1994) in contrast to the United States where the national examination appeared over a decade later (2005). Among the conditions that favoured large-scale use of the OSCE were smaller numbers of Canadian graduates, a less litigious climate in Canada, and control of medical education by a smaller number of medical organizations. Participants cited the administrative and political skills of Richard Reznick (a surgeon from Toronto) and Dale Dauphinee (an internist from Montreal) in the early implementation of the Medical Council of Canada OSCE. Implementation of the first national OSCE was of interest to inventors of simulation technologies, to psychometricians and to simulated and standardized patients. But none of these groups alone had the management expertise to mount what would be a multi-site, human resource-intense and fiscally-demanding national examination. While those involved in assessment in the United States would run experiments and pilot tests for years, and while the UK would delay implementation for more than a decade, Reznick and Dauphinee led a group of people determined to see an OSCE implemented as soon as possible. In his interview, Reznick recalled advising the committee to "remember the exam is going to be very different in a decade…." He added, "we don't have to do it perfectly the first time, we just have to get things started". Dale Dauphinee, Executive Director of the Medical Council of Canada, was noted by many to be a skilled "politician", "administrator" and "leader". Other interviewees confirmed that Reznick, Dauphinee and others who led the development of an OSCE at the MCC tolerated uncertainty to a much greater degree than, for example, the National Board of Medical Examiners in the US who continued to study the idea until implementing it in 2005.

What Reznick brought to the process was labelled a "commitment to implementation" and a "drive to deal with" what he called the "road blocks to production" of the first OSCE. Once in the hands of the MCC OSCE test committee, the priorities for mounting the first national OSCE were not so much academic as "operational". While the first few years did provide an opportunity for invention and a certain degree of research, within a year or two, the focus was on quality control, logistics and efficiency of administration. According to several informants who observed the MCC OSCE development, the Council took "tight control of all data output" and one described a senior administrator at the MCC as "not wanting any academic data to come out of it". Reznick recalled that there was contention over "what we call today intellectual property". He also noted that there were disagreements about publishing. Other participants in my research, who had been involved in the MCC OSCE development, also recalled that the work of the committee was affected by a "bureaucratic" approach in which all questions and all the protocols were carefully reviewed and approved by many levels of staff. The atmosphere was noted to be strikingly different than a medical school.

7.212 Conflicts between Production and Assessment as an Academic Activity

One of the American informants told me that the needs of organizations to mount large-scale tests were in conflict with the academic interests of those who created and studied the technologies on which the examinations would be based. This informant said, "I am going to say something politically incorrect. I think there were some incredibly smart people in this area who were very outspoken, and these people were not involved in the final decision making process for how performance-based assessment was going to be used for licensure". According to informants, the need to subsume academic interests to political goals and to "control" academic work also became an issue for the National Board of Medical Examiners. They grappled with controlling the risk of political or legal fallout from the implementation of a national OSCE that was not supported in all quarters. The development of bureaucratic processes related to performance assessment was part of a shift of OSCE examinations from an academic activity to one of production. Legal and pragmatic considerations became more important than research questions, and the expertise needed to deal with these issues was more administrative than academic.

How did individuals adjust to this shift? As I have noted, Robyn Tamblyn, now a researcher at McGill University, left work with the MCC early for other projects. Arthur Rothman and Gerry Colliver, two psychometricians who had published OSCE research for years, continued to undertake psychometric studies by taking advantage of the opportunities offered by large numbers of candidates and large banks of data. But even these opportunities receded. As people drifted away -- first the innovators, then the researchers and finally even some of the psychometricians, the large organizations moved the examination into the hands of managers and administrators who were less likely to have clinical or academic backgrounds. These changes heralded the dominance of the production discourse related to OSCEs.

A large-scale production model calls for efficiency. However, Reznick recalled that efficiency was challenged at the development committee level. In his words, "a lot of people felt that our snippet version, particularly the five-minute patient encounter, was a bit too trivial". He recalled that Howard Barrows was among the opponents. Reznick told me that the decision was made that shorter cases were sufficient to detect "who knows their stuff and who doesn't". He also noted that this was a decision about efficiency. Referring to the OSCE production scenario, he commented that "a lot of this was generated because of money". Reznick's choice of language in describing the original MCC pilot OSCE illustrated the degree to which the OSCE was already embedded in a discourse of production by the early 1990s. He said, "We had to get things so it was going to be economically feasible, and hence a four or five hour band of testing and being able to test two cohorts in one day became central to running the operation. You had to see it in those days -- it was like command central. It didn't matter what city -- we had phones ringing, adjudication links across the entire country, with frantic calls coming in -- 'We don't know how to interpret this. What do you do with that? How do you answer this?' -- I mean we basically created a command centre for the exam".

7.123 Assessment as a Bureaucratic Activity

The rewards of this project for Reznick and others partly arose from the dimensions of the "operation". Said Reznick, "Oh, it was tremendously exciting. It really was.

Each year we had 500 doctors and a 1000 patients, 1600 students; I mean it's a big enterprise...but it was hugely exciting". But as the experience moved from an innovation to a routinized set of activities, it began to hold less and less appeal. Reznick recalled, "I felt that I was in charge [at the beginning]. Obviously as things matured, I became less and less in charge and more and more people took charge of things". For a while, he said that he continued to stay involved because he felt that he had "an obligation" to do so, but eventually he moved on and left most of the decisions to a host of committees, managers and administrative staff.

A similar history played out at the National Board of Medical Examiners in the US. Danny Klass, the internist from Winnipeg, was recruited in the early 1990s to oversee the national performance-based examination for all US medical graduates. Klass, like Reznick spent as much time dealing with political and operational issues as with research or other academic concerns as the NBME prepared to launch the new massive testing operation. Although initially a magnet for innovators and researchers interested in performance assessment, the NBME too began to discourage publications and academic work arising from the OCSE pilot testing. As issues of "security", "defensibility" and "operations" became priorities, Klass found out that his preferred model of many small testing centres would not be accepted. When he left the NBME, the OSCE-type exam that he had worked on so many years to implement was getting close to reality. However, it would ultimately come to life inside massive testing centres that ran day and night and were a long way from the medical schools where students trained. Klass had argued that huge testing structures risked depersonalizing the examination process and losing the authenticity that made performance testing attractive in the first place. Speaking of the patients trained to play the roles, in an allusion to the manufacturing model, he worried that "if you created a sausage factory, you get sausages". Participants other than Klass also expressed concern that once an institution becomes predominantly focused on production, those with an orientation to innovation, research or the links between performance assessment and learning, drift away.

The production discourse and the associated role of test administrator can clearly be seen at large testing organizations such as the Medical Council of Canada and the National Board of Medical Examinations. But the discourse is not a phenomenon of large institutions only. The production model is also visible at the medical school level. Jean Ker in Dundee and Anja Robb in Toronto both saw the production discourse filtering into the medical school environment. Ker noted that with the evolution of medical education and assessment in the direction of more structured programs, "you have to put in all these management layers for it to function and you lose some of the innovation and disruption". Increased bureaucratic control and regulation, for Ker, are hallmarks of the shift from a focus on the teaching and learning to a more production-oriented model of assessment. This change, she noted, affects the working environment for faculty teachers who have less room for control and creativity as process and hierarchies become more rigid. Robb also commented on the significant shift from creative roles to administrative functions with the growth of high-stakes testing. Ker further associated the phenomena of bureaucratization and hierarchy with gender, observing that male faculty in particular create models of management that foster growth, hierarchical power and control. She noted that "people will talk to me about my 'empire' and I say 'I don't have an empire', I'm here as a 'guardian'. I'm here to ensure that our students get the best education they possibly can". But Ker mused that one will be a more successful academic if one does create, promote and institutionalize one's creations. Robb agreed and talked about her discomfort with the importance given to proliferating job titles.

In summary, in the early days of creation and implementation of big-scale OSCEs, physicians with skills in management took up leadership roles. These included Richard Reznick and Dale Dauphinee at the Medical Council of Canada, Paul Grand'Maison and Joelle Lescop at the College of Family Physicians of Quebec, Gerry Whelan at the Education Commission on Foreign Medical Graduates and Danny Klass at the National Board of Medical Examiners. But once these examinations were in place, the day to day running of these exams moved to professional full-time administrative staff. Thus the discourse of production created the opportunity for some individuals -- mostly men -- to utilize their leadership and management skills. They arrived in these positions because they had legitimacy from previous medical and academic roles and they left having gained even more legitimacy. As I shall discuss below, at the other end of the spectrum, the paid labour force that made the large-scale OSCE possible was made up of administrators and standardized patients, most of whom were women.

7.22 Labour

7.221 Standardized Patient Trainers

As the OSCE was adopted on a larger and larger scale within medical schools and by large testing organizations, the roles that individuals from the standardized patient world could occupy became more circumscribed. As I have detailed above, by the 1990s, the transformation of the role of "simulated patient" that had arisen in the 1960s, to the role of "standardized patient" associated with the rising psychometric discourse, was nearly complete. As "standardized patients programs" (almost never called "simulated patient programs" after the 1980s) become involved in pilot testing and preparation for national OSCE examinations, they often had to put aside their creative efforts in simulation in order to meet the demands of standardized examinations. Smee and others emphasized that not everyone liked this change.

One aspect of the institutionalization of performance-based testing was the training and coordination of a large number of standardized patient activities in an organized and systematic fashion. In a manner that fit well with the principles of scientific management, the role of Standardized Patient Trainer became institutionalized and formalized. SP trainers were responsible for management of standardized patient programs, including human resources and financial issues; training and development; monitoring of performance consistency and quality; and negotiating the interface between "professional consultants" and "content experts" (physicians) and the testing administrative staff and managers discussed above. In the largest of institutions, the Standardized Patient Trainer was herself a manager. In a medical school, she was often an administrator, although in some cases after about the year 2000, she might also have a faculty appointment.

Because of their closeness to the working conditions, professional development and personal lives of standardized patients, trainers often adopted the role of advocates and set the stage for what is now a growing movement (particularly in the US) toward the professionalization of standardized patients. Standardized patient trainers taking up these functions became conversant in the language of labour negotiations,

191

professional organization, standard setting, governance, human resources and finance. The need to attend to the "business" aspects of standardized patient work, whether in a medical school or in a testing organization, was part of the uptake of the discourse of production.

Gayle Gliva-McConvey was the president of the Association of Standardized Patient Educators when I interviewed her. Gliva-McConvey had written in 1995 that "[w]ith the growth in demand for SPs, a new occupation has emerged – that of standardized patient" (Woodward & Gliva-McConvey, 1995, p. 418). She was one of several participants who argued that standardized patients are part of an "emerging profession". I have described in Chapter 5 the precursor roles that evolved into the "professional" standardized patient starting almost 40 years ago with the women who acted as largely passive "models" in the classroom. With the emergence of psychometric discourse, there was a change in the role of simulated patient to standardized patient. The SP became an element of a process of psychometric testing. With the subsequent rise of a discourse of production, standardized patients became essential labour in running large-scale OSCEs.

With the emergence of large-scale testing institutions, new issues such as job security and professional identity, not previously given much attention by part-time and volunteer women SPs came to the fore. Sociologist Anne Witz (1992) has written cogently about the processes by which "new" professions emerge and the strategies by which they shape the nature and legitimacy of their work. More specifically, Witz has studied the gendered nature of processes of professionalization. It is important to note that standardized patients and standardized patient trainers are over 80 percent women. On the other hand, as noted previously, most educational psychometricians discussed in the last chapter and most of the senior administrators in testing organizations are men. Thus the efforts of these groups to achieve authority and legitimacy are clearly gendered.

7.222 The Professionalization of SPs

Professionalization of SPs is linked to production discourse in a clearer way than it ever was with performance or psychometric discourse. As I discussed in chapter 5, in early performance discourse, the only role for women SPs was as teaching and assessment tools. Later, psychometric discourse opened the door a crack for a few SPs to re-train as psychometricians, but this was a long, arduous road and one taken by only a few women such as Robyn Tamblyn. As the work of SPs gained more legitimacy in both universities and in testing organizations. Linda Perkowski, for example, moved from being a Standardized Patient Trainer and Program Director to become Associate Dean at the University of Minnesota. Sydney Smee became the manager of the Medical Council of Canada OSCE. Gayle Gliva-McConvey created and became the president of a national association of SPs (ASPE), and Devra Cohen became Manager of the Morchand Centre (a collaboration of eight medical schools in Manhattan), and later also president of ASPE. I will consider the careers of these women in some detail to illustrate both the possibilities and the constraints created for them by production discourse.

Beginning her career at McMaster, Sydney Smee, along with many others of today's leaders in the standardized patient world, pursued a trajectory that led her in the 1990s to become national manager of the Medical Council of Canada OSCEs. Here she has major responsibilities for the nature of and running of the Canadian medical certification examinations. At the beginning of her career it was far from evident that she would pursue such a career. Standardized patient colleagues, such as Gayle Gliva-McConvey, figured prominently in her account of her career. Gliva-McConvey, with whom Smee worked over 20 years ago at McMaster, recalled meeting Smee. "I was at my office and I looked up, and there's this sort of girl in construction boots, blue jeans, lumberjack shirt, long hair, 16 years old, wanting a job. And that was it" she recalled. Gliva McConvey gave Smee her first job. Smee herself recalled, "I was in high school. My mother and I filled in and my sister, my father and mother did a mother-daughter role around abortion, for an OBGYN conference work group that was running at Mac. That's where I met Gayle. I had a lot of fun doing that, so it became my part-time job through high school and through university". She was so drawn to being an SP that she recalled, "I'd skip school to go into work -- with my mother's permission!" Smee didn't go to university for several years after high school, which gave her an opportunity to do more work with the Standardized Patient Program, including covering Gliva-McConvey's maternity leave.

Smee also worked as a gynaecological teaching associate, recalling that it was "a powerful teaching opportunity" and that she had a good degree of control as the teacher. "I just looked at one of those terrified faces and thought, 'wow, you've got a problem, I don't'". This contrasts with Smee's observations about her sense of powerlessness as a standardized patient around behaviour verging on abusiveness that occurred in a few teaching situations when physicians were present. The experience of a greater sense of power and control during a pelvic exam as compared to a routine cardiac exam is remarkable and illustrates that power and control is taken up by the physician in the one case, and the authorized role of the patient as teacher or as model in the other. Reflecting on the effects of power and being an SP, Smee observed that "a basic premise with patient instructors is that when you're teaching you have total control. In an OSCE you can't". For this and other reasons, she was attracted to Massachusetts where Paula Stillman was developing her patient instructors. However, by that point Stillman was moving into more psychometric measures and so Smee returned to Toronto where she worked part-time with the Standardized Patient Program run by Anja Robb. Finally, she was hired to work on the Medical Council of Canada's OSCE project. Smee then rose through the administrative structure at the Medical Council, her role growing in tandem with the importance of the national OSCE.

Smee was identified by many key informants as a key person in the development of OSCEs on a large scale. Both her interview and the way in which she is seen by others in the field illustrated the influence of the discourse of production. She told me that "by and large people don't argue over whether you could or should use standardized patients anymore; now they argue over cost". Her concerns were about the efficiency of production of the OSCE and she called her work "our end of the business". However, she was aware of the effects, both positive and negative, of power that is taken up by institutions linked to the production of large scales examinations.

As she works for SPs, Smee told me she tries to use her position to advance their interests. In her words, "it's mattered a lot to me to have connections with people like Gayle [Gliva-McConvey] and Linda [Perkowski] as an organization that hires a lot of trainers. You feel some responsibility to promote peoples' participation, to support the

development of – I don't know if it's a profession – but it is certainly an occupation".
From her vantage point at the Medical Council, she also has a sense of how to gain
legitimacy. She told me, "I see it as my role to encourage [SPs] to be members of the
Association of Standardized Patient Educations (ASPE), to think about doing
research, to go to the Ottawa conference". Further, she tries to use her position at the
Medical Council to bring together standardized patient trainers. Her goal, she said, is
"to promote the professionalism of the group". As Smee's career progressed at the
Medical Council of Canada, however, she moved farther away from the teaching
environment of medical schools. Asked to characterize her job today, she called
herself a "manager" in the field of "medical licensure", defining it as an
administrative role.

For Gail Gliva-McConvey, before any professionalization project could become
possible, it was necessary to alter the perception of the subject position of the
standardized patient, from a depersonalized assessment "tool" to an embodied
individual possessing ability, choice and agency. This reconstitution of the nature of
the standardized patient was signalled by an article that appeared in the literature in
1995. Coauthored with a female PhD-educator when she was a standardized patient
program director, the paper not only described the personal abilities, struggles and
impacts of work as a standardized patient, it also declared that "a new occupation"
had emerged (Woodward & Gliva-McConvey, 1995, p. 418). Similar articles
focussing on the impact of the work of standardized patients have appeared since,
such as a paper by McNaughton et al. (1999) that explored the emotional effects of
playing challenging roles. McNaughton is now also pursuing a PhD.

Since the publication of the 1995 paper, Gliva-McConvey has been leading a process
that she hopes will bring greater acceptance and autonomy for standardized patients.
Now Director of the Theresa A. Thomas Professional Skills Teaching and Assessment
Centre at Eastern Virginia Medical School in Norfolk Virginia and President of The
Association of Standardized Patient Educators, Gliva-McConvey represents a
generation of women who began as part-time standardized patients, moved into
training and, rather than trying to advance through positions in research, with testing
organizations or in administration, chose to directly advance the professionalization
project of standardized patients. As noted, Gliva-McConvey started her career as the

coordinator of the Standardized Patient Program at McMaster University in the 1980s when she worked with Howard Barrows. At that time, the discourse was moving from classroom applications of standardized patients to large scale assessment and research applications. In her words, these new opportunities were a "nice extension of the use of standardized patients, which, of course got more exposure of our standardized patients, and more work for our standardized patients… [and] the program grew as a result".

7.223   The Association of Standardized Patient Educators

In recent years, Gliva-McConvey and others such as Cohen, Perkowski, Robb and Adamo have carried further the project to advance the career of standardized patients by creating opportunities for networking. First there was a special interest group at the Association of American Medical Colleges (AAMC) which "provided a forum for SP educators". Then in the 1990s, the AAMC made changes to its structure such that the SP special interest group was discontinued. With the demise of the special interest group at the US national medical education meeting, Gliva-McConvey and others created their own organization, the Association of Standardized Patient Educators (ASPE). Today, she told me, "we have over 400 members. We are international! There is North America of course, the Netherlands, we've got Spain, we've got Germany, and we've got Korea. Where else? Britain. No one from France yet [but] it keeps expanding". Graceanne Adamo is another leader in the SP field who is Director of Clinical Skills, Teaching and Assessment at the National Capital Area Medical Simulation Centre. Having worked with the ECFMG and the NBME, she has written about the need for SPs to advance as a profession though development of formal organizational structures, and called ASPE the "specialist professional organization" (Adamo, 2003).

Both Gliva-McConvey and Devra Cohen, in their interviews, provided details about the professionalization project for the SP association, including the development of a charter, membership criteria and standards of practice. These elements are common to emerging professional groups as part of the effort to stake a turf over which they have control (Witz, 1992; Gieryn, 1983). Often linked to issues of safety, the invoking of standards of practice is a particularly effective way of using discourse to enact "closure" on the domain of a new profession from "unprofessional outsiders". Standards of practice, held in place by definitions of professional competence or scope of practice and required training programs, certification and examinations, help define the boundaries of professional control. The boundaries are useful both to guard and protect areas of practice that are deemed to be unique to the profession, and to extrude areas of practice that are no longer desirable as part of practice.

Cohen told me that, during her term as president of ASPE, "one of the things I really pushed on the agenda was putting together a certificate program". Cohen saw the need to develop certification but also education for members in areas such as statistics and curriculum development. She saw one of the missions of ASPE as "to help develop its membership". A key element of professionalization, she argued, is the creation of a hierarchy of different SP jobs. She saw a need "to start defining different levels of competency of the job. For instance a trainer, versus a coordinator, versus a standardized or simulated patient educator, versus a director". Gliva-McConvey also argued that ASPE has a role to play in professionalizing SP work. She said, "we have an annual meeting but we've moved now from just being a forum to starting to develop some standards. I'm the chair of the Standards of Practice Committee". When I asked her to elaborate on what she meant by standards she said, "we'll start developing some standards of practice guidelines. There are no checks and balances, so one of the hazards of interacting with a bad standardized patient is that people start disbelieving in the methodology. You can have one bad standardized patient interaction and it takes you three or four more to get rid of that bad taste in your mouth". Expanding on the role of standards in raising the profile of the profession, she noted that "we're thinking of certification in the future. There needs to be a body that we're policing [showing] that we're responsible for ourselves".

This last point is rather important because it was followed with "before someone else does". Here Gliva-McConvey clearly illustrated the role of power in the evolution and control of the profession and the very real threat in her mind that control might be lost. When I asked her, "Who's the someone else?" she identified the large testing organizations. In her words, "the Medical Council and the National Board are recognized as being pretty influential in medical education. Of course they're using

197

standardized patients [and] so we want to make sure that we please ourselves rather than someone like the National Board or somebody else".

7.224   Gender and Standardized Patients

The importance of working with and developing the careers of other women by creating opportunities for work, teaching and assessment was a frequent refrain in my interviews with women who work as standardized patients and trainers. By contrast, I would find no paper or any reference to this form of mentorship and support in the published standardized patient or OSCE literature. Wallace's (1997) original history of SPs spoke of the "great innovators" who developed standardized patients -- all of whom are physicians, but did not deal with the mentoring of standardized patients by their peers. While a few articles have addressed the personal side of the job, such as McNaughton et al. (1999) and Woodward (1995), both of these explored the physical and emotional effects on the people who play roles as standardized patients. Today there are still no articles that capture the developmental role of women leaders who have pushed forward to create opportunities for a generation of standardized patients. Devra Cohen talked about the difficulties SPs face in finding mentorship and support. As a faculty member with neither a PhD nor an MD Cohen, who like many SP leaders has a master's degree, found it very difficult initially to find colleagues and advocates in the University. Eventually she found a group of women faculty who supported each other and discussed issues such as careers and promotion. She also associated herself with Jerry Colliver, a psychometrician, who helped her gain legitimacy in the eyes of her own university by teaching her psychometric analysis, offering to help with her research projects and involving her as an author on publications.

And yet, among the participants in this study, there was a strong awareness of the gendered nature of the work and of the struggles related to labour issues. Sydney Smee explained why most SPs are women and then likened the role of standardized patient to a casual lover. She told me, "I think it's a reflection that there's often very little money and it wasn't regular hours so that it was women who were available to do a job that didn't have to support anybody, or we got by on very little money". She elaborated that, "being an SP for sometimes very demanding, emotional roles -- the students would have this wonderful experience and they would all go off and get coffee and I would go home. You can start to feel used. If you were being dramatic about it, it would be a one-night stand. They would go off – you guys are all happy and I am left sitting here".

Robyn Tamblyn explained the female domination of standardized patient work as a phenomenon of recruitment and demographics, arguing that women in the 20 to 40 age group have been more available than men. She said that "when you recruit standardized patients, if you're looking for the age range 20 through 50, there are women who are doing part-time work, volunteer work, or they're at home looking after the kids. And they're available during the day when you need standardized patients. Men, on the other hand, are working, and are not available during those times when you need standardized patients.... It's very difficult recruiting any male between 20 and 40". Anja Robb, Director of the University of Toronto Standardized Patient Program, added the dimension of acceptability of the work undertaken by SPs to account for the low pay. She explained, "we're starting to get more men, but we're still overwhelmingly a female job. If you think about my own past to this point, I'm wondering how many men could have afforded to work six jobs a year at $8 an hour as I did when I started. You know, I'm married and I wouldn't starve if I made $200 a year. Our society still hasn't evolved that far, and I think that men in general have to be more conscious about establishing careers and earning money". Diana Tabak echoed this pointing out that "these are all people who need money to support themselves". She noted that SP teaching pays much less than assessment and added that, although she doesn't know of any SP who, given a choice, would choose to work in assessment over teaching, the decision is, in the end "economic".

7.225 SP Unionization and Funding Issues in North America

All of these women, along with other participants, cited increasing professionalization as an antidote to the use of women as a "reserve army of labour". SP leader priorities now are to consolidate their role and improve their position. What is striking is the degree to which the discourse associated with this professionalization is one of business, labour relations, working conditions and other aspects of business and capital linked to the discourse of production. Robb argued that "we are no longer fighting for legitimacy in the work we do. Now we are looking at ways to improve what we do, collaborate better in what we do.... So yes, we are professionalizing: we are no longer just the appendage to medical faculty to run their research". McKinley at the ECFMG, expressed certainty that standardized patients will unionize. She said, "folks are creating guidelines for work conditions – but you can't constrain them – they're people!" Noting the role of "human factors" such as stress, she argued that there will be a "fee and benefit structure", that there will be "big employment and fee issues" and that as a group SPs will soon address such issues as buying group insurance. She noted the importance of attending to the health, well being and positive attitude of SPs as part of maintaining the high quality of their work, and good working relations. In Canada, Tabak explained that the University of Toronto SPs are part of the Steel Workers of America. This, she said, has been "very beneficial for those of us who are on staff", but noted that "there are no benefits for the majority of SPs who are casual, part-time employees. Across the border in the US, Cohen also noted the economic reasons that most SPs remain contract workers. As she explained, "if they were part-time, you would have to pay for health benefits and a lot of other things that will make them completely cost ineffective".

Danny Klass, once at the National Board of Medical Examiners, thought it was likely that SPs there would unionize. He argued, however, that this is unlikely to become a problem for the NBME because it is almost the only large-scale employer of SPs in the US. As he remarked, "you pay what you can pay and the union ... wouldn't be an effective union if it just destroyed the industry". Co-incidentally, Klass had just returned from giving the keynote address for the annual ASPE meeting when I interviewed him. He told me that "here is a great group of people who have really boot-strapped a profession. I think they do great work and need to be recognized as professionals. There should be a school and degrees and all that kind of stuff". Jack Boulet at the ECFMG agreed that the SP group needs to professionalize by obtaining master's degrees in education and measurement. However, he noted that the same forces that led SPs to replace MD examiners might in turn lead to the replacement of SPs, if technologies such as computer simulations ever become more efficient and lower cost than SP simulations.

Devra Cohen described another aspect of the economics of SP work that makes it tenuous. Not only are most SPs part-time or contract workers, but the larger SP programs themselves receive little or no funding from their medical schools. According to Cohen, The Morchand Centre in New York, the SP program in Toronto and the SP program run by Gayle Gliva-McConvey in West Virginia, are all responsible for finding their own sustaining funding. She worried that "the portion [of the budget] that is coming from the medical school is actually getting smaller". As a result, Cohen, Robb, Gliva-McConvey and others must become "entrepreneurial" in order for their programs to survive. The Morchand Centre, for example, was created with funding for three years by the Macy Foundation. Their original mission was to bring together eight New York medical schools to help them incorporate SPs and OSCE examinations. They also functioned as a site for much of the development work for the eventual national NBME examination. However, after the first three years, Cohen said she, like other SP program directors, had to search for outside sources of funding. She gave a recent example of offering a contract to provide services to the customer service department of a large health care delivery organization that was "getting a bad reputation for the way in which they treat their patients". She also told me that SP programs increasingly take on contract work from pharmaceutical companies and drug representatives. Finally, Cohen told me, the huge testing corporation, Kaplan, also works with SP programs to develop courses for international medical graduates. Cohen said all of these efforts to seek funds create tensions and so "some people felt threatened". They question whether her organization is "academic or for profit".

The ongoing professionalization of standardized patients in North America was thrown into sharp relief during my interviews in Europe. I have noted in my discussion of the psychometric discourse that Scotland never adopted the term "standardized patient" and continues with the older term "simulated patient". While this represents a rejection of the psychometric discourse, it is also linked to the failure of simulated patients in Scotland to develop their occupation in the direction of a profession, as is occurring in North America. There was no indication of this process taking place in Scotland that I could discover. Whereas Anja Robb at University of Toronto and Gayle Gliva McConvey at East Virginia spoke at length about the professional aspirations for SPs, I was unable to locate such a leader at Dundee. While I was told that there was "some sort of association" of actors who are used for teaching communication skills and ethics, there was a strong sense that it would be unimaginable to have SPs providing the majority of marks for students. Teaching clinical skills in a significant way also seemed unlikely to my Scottish key informants. Said Jean Ker, "certainly never in Scotland do we have somebody on staff who has been a simulated patient". She went on, "I know with the ECFMG it's standardized patients that do the actual marking. I have a problem with that". She described her feeling that while the SP can "give you the patient's perspective" she felt that even if they are health professionals, they are in a conflict because they are simultaneously playing the patient and evaluator. She argued that these are two very different perspectives, which should be kept separate. Important here is her resistance to the conflation of the roles of simulator and of observer -- a distinction that is important for those using a discourse of performance as I have described with links to teaching, learning and feedback. As I have noted above, this distinction disappears as the focus shifts to the imperatives of efficiency in both dollars and personnel that is part of the discourse of production. This distinction was underscored when I asked Ker if she felt that in the US standardized patients were used as assessors in order to emphasize the patient perspective. She responded, "No, I think they're doing it because it's cost effective".

The imperative for cost effectiveness and its implications for SPs are illustrated by the merger that took place during the expansion from the one-site ECFMG examination to the five-site national US exam. At this size of production, efficiencies of scale and cost containment became important issues and one major costs of an OSCE is standardized patients. Thus the costs associated with SP training and work came under scrutiny. Gerry Whelan noted that there was a difference of philosophy between the ECFMG and the NBME. He pointed out that all the trainers at the ECFMG were themselves standardized patients who had worked their way up to the position of trainer at the NBME, however, many of the trainers are not SPs. As Whelan pointed out, the NBME "wanted people with a master's degree". Recently, the role of trainer has come under further scrutiny. A research study presented at the Association of Medical Educators in Europe explored the possibility of removing the trainer altogether and using the internet to have standardized patients train themselves for reasons of cost saving.

Despite all these constraints, women who are standardized patients have, by all accounts, gained more legitimacy and authority in recent years than they had in the 1960s. But arguably any authority that they have won depends to a large degree on their proximity to sources of legitimacy rooted in dominant discourses, and arises much less directly from the standardized patient work itself. Unlike the scientist or the physician, the standardized patient does not work in an area that directly brings prestige.

Danny Klass argued that the real struggle for standardized patients is now economic. There will be "an inevitable loss of a variety of intangibles", he said, when education and testing units get "too big" because "you lose the relationship between the trainer and each individual standardized patient". He noted that the decision of the National Board of Medical Examiners to move to only five very large testing centres in the United States was based on "a question of efficiency" that has pitted economic and educational priorities against one another. The evolution of larger and more rigid corporate structures may present their project with further challenges.

7.3   Institutions and Production Discourse

Based on my analysis of the literature and my visits to institutions in the US, Canada and the UK, I would argue that the discourse of production is much more prominent in the United States than in Canada, and in Canada more than in the United Kingdom. There are several reasons for this, not the least of which is the role of large national institutions in medical education. In the US, the National Board of Medical Examiners has a monopoly on the assessment of all medical graduates and thus wields a great deal of power with other national organizations such as the American Medical Association and educational groups such as the Association of American Medical Colleges (AAMC) and the speciality boards. In effect, medical schools have transferred much of their summative decisions about physician competence to the national organization. At the specialty level, strong boards coordinate national testing and are loosely affiliated across specialty areas. In Canada, there are strong national organizations involved in testing as well, including the Medical Council of Canada at the undergraduate level. The Royal College of Physicians and Surgeons and College of Family Physicians integrate testing at the specialty level. These organizations also have a great deal of power in setting the national agenda for testing and education. If they are slightly less dominant than the NBME, this is perhaps because of the more central role of universities in Canada, and the dispersion of control of testing and licensure through multiple provincial and national agencies. To some degree, the provincial licensure authorities, although they no longer conduct their own examinations, are very active in pushing for certain elements such as the recent emphasis on ethics and communication skills. In the UK, it is not even possible to point to one or a few large testing organizations. There is a Royal College of each specialty and these are only starting to work together on a national framework. There remains no organization that administers a final examination at the end of medical school. Thus, more power remains in the hands of individual medical schools to set examinations and determine the trajectory of their graduates.

In the next section, I explore the nature of the large testing organizations that have become influential in the promulgation of the discourse of production and that have triggered the associated issues of SPs working conditions, professionalization and efficiency of production explored above.

7.31   Medical Council of Canada (MCC)

Sir Thomas Roddick, according to the Medical Council's own history, "pursued his vision of a national medical licensing standard within Canada, through legislation, for over 18 years" (MCC, 2006). His efforts led to the passage of a bill in the Canadian Parliament known as the Canada Medical Act that resulted in the formation of the Medical Council of Canada in 1912. The first national examination for medical graduates was held in Montreal in 1913 (MCC, 2006).

Since that time, the MCC has had as its mission "promoting a uniform standard of qualification to practice medicine for all physicians across Canada" (MCC, 2006). The qualification issued after meeting the standards and passing the examinations of the MCC is called the Licentiate of the Medical Council of Canada (LMCC) and is the primary form of certification that is acceptable to provincial medical regulatory authorities for issuance of a licence to practice medicine. Thus, the activities of the MCC are central to the control of who is able to practice medicine in Canada and who is not. The MCC makes a clear rhetorical link between assessment and quality of medical care -- thus establishing its legitimacy on the basis of examinations. The official vision statement is: "striving for the highest level of medical care for Canadians through excellence in the evaluation of physicians". Arising from this vision, the MCC conducts two national examinations --- a Part 1 written test of knowledge administered at the end of medical school training and a Part 2 OSCE given after 18 months of postgraduate training.

During the 1950s, the MCC formed an alliance with the US National Board of Medical Examiners to use their written tests. Effectively, Canadian certification used an American exam. However, with the formation of the R.S. McLaughlin Examination and Research Center at Laval University and the University of Alberta in 1968, there was a move toward "more Canadian content and eventual repatriation of the examination from the National Board of Medical Examiners" (MCC, 2006). By 1977, the examinations were fully "repatriated" and by 1977 the MCC had developed a new "Evaluating Examination" that was first administered for graduates of foreign medical schools in January 1979. The MCC continues to offer this examination in countries around the world. In 1987, a "Future Directions Task Force" was created by the MCC to explore a new examination that would assess clinical skills and in particular, communication. This led to the development of MCCQE Part II, the national Objective Structured Clinical Examination (OSCE) using standardized patients that was chaired by Richard Reznick and described in detail above.

7.311 Fertile Conditions for the Development of a Large-Scale OSCE

In examining the history of the Medical Council of Canada, it is helpful to put it in the context of the development of other institutions. For example, during the middle of the twentieth century in Canada, specialty medicine and then family medicine were created and led to a new layer of organizations that imposed training requirements and examinations which must be attained before authorization to practice medicine. The creation of the Royal College of Physicians and Surgeons of Canada (RCPSC) in 1929 as a "national, private, non-profit organization" (RCPSC, 2006) was also made possible by an Act of Parliament. That Act specified that the RCPSC would "oversee postgraduate medical education" and thus the College "sets up criteria for the designation of a specialty, develops and defines the educational objectives and national standards for medical, laboratory, and surgical specialties; accredits specialty training programs; and conducts examinations for certificates of qualification" (RCSPC, 2006) . Today, the RCPSC states that it is "an organization of medical specialists dedicated to ensuring the highest standards and quality of health care". The RCPSC calls itself "the voice of specialty care in Canada" that "ensures that the training and evaluation of medical and surgical specialists in 60 specialties and two special programs attain the highest standards" (RCPSC, 2006). From the beginning it was the role of the College to "act and speak out in support of the most appropriate context for the practice of specialty care and the best patient care". Its mission overlaps with the Medical Council of Canada. However, the RCPSC was never authorized to act as a licensing or disciplinary body thus has directed its efforts towards a mission that is "educational and dedicated to setting standards" (RCPSC, 2006). Consistent with this direction, the RCPSC gradually evolved distinct processes for the education and certification of a rising group of specialties. While in 1929 there were only two specialty qualifications (in general medicine and general surgery), by 1937, the College offered specialty qualifications in seven areas: dermatology, ophthalmology, otolaryngology, paediatrics, diagnostic radiology, therapeutic radiology, and urology. Gradually more specialty qualifications were created and College now recognizes 60 specialty and subspecialty qualifications (RCSPC, 2006).

Another important institution in the Canadian medical landscape is the College of Family Physicians of Canada (CFPC), established in 1954 as "a national voluntary organization of family physicians that makes continuing medical education of its members mandatory" (CFPC, 2006). The College lists among its missions that it aims to "improve the health of Canadians by promoting high standards of medical education and care in family practice". Like the RCPSC, the CFPC took on roles in accreditation of education programs, advocacy and, as well, the creation of new examinations. According to their website, "since 1969, 12,500 physicians have written the exam and more than 70 percent of all members have achieved certification and now use the CCFP designation" (CFPC, 2006). Rhetorically, the evolution of this body also overlapped with the jurisdiction of the MCC and the RCPSC in its examination functions and has pursued a certain amount of competition with them.

While in 1912, when the Medical Council of Canada was created, a medical degree plus the Council examinations qualified a doctor for practice, by the end of the twentieth century, the MCC exams qualified one only as part of a package that would eventually lead to licensure, but which also required success on either the speciality or family medicine examinations. Thus, part of the Medical Council's interest in development of their national OSCE was to strengthen its mandate at a time when there were questions about the importance of a national test of knowledge. In proposing the national OSCE, the Medical Council argued that the new examination would be a nationally portable qualification. Richard Reznick told me that what was achieved actually fell short of that goal. He explained that "a lot of people had a lot of antibodies for this exam, because they felt…that it didn't do what it was set up to do and that was to create a set of qualifications that were totally portable and meaningful. And the reason that happened is because the family doctors won their longstanding battle to develop a speciality of their own. So part of it is around the politics and then the money".

In this analysis are recognizable elements of production discourse. The attention to politics, economic concerns, labour relations and competition meant that the OSCE, in this environment, served a new and different purpose than when it was employed in teaching institutions. No longer was the OSCE simply a tool for education as a part of the iterative performance-feedback loop that characterized the discourse of performance. Nor was it just a tool used primarily to convert human performance into numbers as it became within the psychometric discourse. Now it was an instrument linked to institutional goals that had political and economic meaning; more specifically, it became linked to the professionalization project of physicians including the dream of "global standards of competence" (Stern, Friedman Ben-David, Norcini, Wojtczak & Schwartz, 2006). As large institutions tried to achieve these goals using the language of production, the OSCEs the created took on the coloration of this discourse.

Within production discourse, attention to the quality of the "product" and addressing the needs of "stakeholders" are common rhetorical constructions. Thus, among the many arguments used to adopt a large-scale national OSCE in Canada, protection of the public is one of the more common ones. Smee noted that, "from a lay public point of view, there always should have been something like an OSCE....[T]heir assumption is that doctors do get tested that way". The students I interviewed in Canada talked to me about the MCC in terms of fairness in relationship to multiple observations. Said one, "I much prefer being examined by six to 12 examiners". Interestingly, neither of the Canadian students had ever experienced any other kind of performance-based, certification examination. In response to my question about large-scale OSCE examinations, one of the students suggested that they serve to "inspire confidence from the public, knowing that every doctor in the country has passed the same examination". However, another student suggested that the MCC OSCE was created "for historical reasons" and yet another called it "an examination without a purpose". That student added, "I'm not sure that the doctors who graduated before the advent of OSCEs were bad doctors or incompetent doctors", arguing that the highly standardized OSCE, with its many short cases, actually "allows you to study a little less deeply".

7.321   Education Commission on Foreign Medical Graduates/National Board of Medical Examiners (ECFMG/NBME)

7.321   A Corporate Merger

In the last chapter the evolution of the American Education Commission on Foreign Medical Graduates was outlined. Gerry Whelan, the current Director of the ECFMG, argued that the reason for the adoption of large scale OSCEs in the US was that "with the advent of technology, there was a general concern that basic clinical skills were being neglected". This is, of course, a familiar part of the performance discourse. However, the direction this took within medical schools and where it would go when the ECFMG merged with the National Board of Medical Examiners were very different. While medical schools adopted a performance discourse to implement simulations for teaching and assessment, the ECFMG and NBME implemented OSCEs because medical school, in Whelan's words, "could not be trusted" to sufficiently assess performance themselves. In the case of the ECFMG, the problem was one of assessing the quality and outcome of attending medical schools outside of the US, but later the NBME would extend this argument to include a lack of confidence in American medical schools as well. In the 1990s, the ECFMG

implemented a large OSCE called the CSA (Clinical Skills Assessment) for all
international medical graduates wishing to enter the American Medical Education
system. Success on the CSA was the only route to access to America residency
training. Later, after the year 2000, when the ECFMG was merged with the NBME,
the same examination (the name was changed to the CS) was made mandatory for all
graduates of US medical schools.

The implementation was not easy. As Whelan recalled, while "US medical schools
have always tolerated the USMLE" [United States Medical Licensing Examination],
"they were not at all happy with the CS. They were not supportive. They felt they
should be able to assess themselves". Whelan noted that the American Medical
Association protested the implementation of the NBME's OSCE-type examination on
behalf of medical students who were also opposed. Whelan's analysis is that the
medical schools felt that this examination was 'intruding on their jurisdiction".

I have previously described how the national implementation of an OSCE was a long
time coming in the US. Many of the same people who worked on the Medical Council
of Canada OSCE consulted to the ECFMG and the NBME. There had already been
many research papers published related to OSCEs since the 1970s. As I described, the
early papers linked to the discourse of performance elaborated means of
implementing OSCEs at medical schools. These papers often addressed the role of the
OSCE within curricula and its links to teaching and learning. Later, as the
psychometric discourse became more prominent, issues of reliability, validity and
generalizability came to dominate. However, as attention turned to the possibility of a
much larger-scale national examination, a production discourse took hold, and the
issues of concern changed. For example, working with the ECFMG, Paula Stillman
moved away from the issues that had preoccupied her in developing patient
instructors and conducted a study entitled, "Is Test Security an Issue in a Multi-
Station Clinical Assessment?" (Stillman et al., 1991). In the same year, Stillman
collaborated with Miriam Friedman and Al Sutnick from the ECFMG and John
Norcini from the NBME to explore the feasibility of the OSCE as an assessment of
English proficiency of foreign medical graduates (Friedman et al., 1991).

The language of papers emerging from those working with the ECFMG/NBME was decidedly more "operational" throughout the 1990s as they prepared the massive new examination. Stillman wrote a review of the use of standardized patients in 1993 concluding that "further research must be done before SPs can be used for high-stakes certifying and licensing examinations". The ECFMG continued its research which was summarized in papers such as those written by Sutnick et al. (1993; 1994). Joint research projects between the two organizations started to appear in the late 1990s (e.g. Ben-David et al., 1999). Research would continue in earnest on expansion of this examination for all US graduates until it was finally implemented in 2005. This large-scale merger can be seen as a step in the corporatization and globalization of the American model of examination in medicine. The central influence of the new organization in exporting technologies and standards of assessment around the world can be seen, as well as the shaping effect of having only one route of access for medical professionals who wish to gain certification in the United States.

I visited the merged institution and interviewed a number of employees, both current and past. This merger could be compared to corporate mergers that took place in the private business sector throughout the 1990s. It was linked to discourses that characterize neo-liberal economics which include such words as "efficiency", "productivity", "economies of scale" and the like. Like many mergers, it also involved a fairly difficult marginalization of distinct cultures. I found that significant tensions remain between individuals who still identify themselves with one organization or the other. For example, many of the ECFMG staff members refer to the NBME as "the folks up the street" in a way that makes it clear that the National Board is "somewhere else". On the other hand, in a public lecture I attended, one of the senior administrators of the NBME talked about the period "after the ECFMG went off line".

It was the development of the national OSCE that led to the merger. While the ECFMG ran its large-scale OSCE for all international medical graduates after 1996, the NBME was only conducting a national written examination for American medical graduates. Bringing the two organizations together would theoretically allow them to combine their strength for the mammoth task of assessing 25,000 American medical graduates each year with an OSCE. This scale of OSCE, in terms of financing, human resources and political ramifications greatly exceeded anything that had come before. But, the NBME was a much larger organization than the ECFGM and was the more dominant partner in the new merged institution. One of the people interviewed noted that the shift in discourses was related to changes in who held power in the new merged institution, explaining that "culturally, at the ECFMG, clinicians outnumbered psychometricians. There were three full time physicians and two psychometricians at the ECFMG while, at the NBME, they are mostly psychometricians -- there are only two MDs and a horde of possibly 20 to 30 psychometricians".

7.322 The Shift to Production Discourse

As noted many times, in the hands of the National Board of Medical Examiners, the OSCE underwent over a decade of development, refinement and testing that built on, but differed from the work done by the ECFMG. At the NBME, the process was overseen by the large group of psychometricians more familiar initially with the large scale multiple choice tests administered for many years by the Board. This shifted the OSCE considerably and, as Gliva-McConvey put it, "the National Board says, this is the methodology. Now it's called a methodology, not just an innovative teaching tool: now it's a methodology".

As the NBME moved from a research focus to a mode of production, there was a commensurate shift in discourse. Danny Klass, formerly in charge of OSCE development at the NBME, explained that "mantra for us at the National Board was always that we had three issues to deal with. First validity, second reliability and third feasibility". He explained that the first two -- reliability and validity -- had been dealt with in a number of "small scale projects and other people's experience". According to Klass, the focus shifted to issues of feasibility for the implementation of a large-scale national examination: "Once you know it can be done, there is an imperative to do it. The only reason not to do it would be because it's too expensive or that it's politically unacceptable. What else can there be? You know it reliable; you know its valid so there's got to be something – feasibility. So that's where all the attention ended up going".

7.323   The Problem of "Demographics"

There are several implications of the corporatization of OSCEs and the shift of focus from examination as a tool for feedback about performance to examination as institutional product. First, one issue I heard about repeatedly was euphemistically called "demographics". For the ECFMG staff, there had previously been an emphasis on dealing with issues of ethno-racial diversity among their patient cases, which I discussed in the last chapter. This was central for the ECFMG, given its orientation to the testing of international medical graduates. But for the NBME, as discussed, too much "variability" in cases was a problem for statistical analysis. As might be expected, as the discourse shifted from more "pure" psychometric concerns to issues of production, the standardization of patient cases and of their demographics were connected to the efficiency of examination implementation and analysis. As production discourse replaced psychometric discourse, standardized patients needed to be similar, not just to "eliminate variance" but also to "streamline the process" of training and to "make it more efficient". One staff member at the ECFMG told me that the removal of patient demographics became a problem. As this informant explained it, "I look at the cases and I see stereotypical Anglo-Saxon names. I think we need to break out of all the notions of race and culture and religion. We fought really hard to break out of those specifications, but it is evolving from a notion that it was very important, to something else". Reflecting on the merger, this informant said that the "measurement folks wanted standardization of, for example, skin colour [seeing it as] as a feature to control during the exam. If they could use clones, they would use clones".

I had heard similar comments in Canada in relation to the Medical Council of Canada examination. Sydney Smee told me that she worried that with large examinations there is a tendency to "homogenize". She spoke about her concerns related to the "message" that large examinations can send. She concluded that "for our OSCE and recruiting across the country, we tend to end up presenting a very white middle class section. There are hidden messages and hidden consequences to what we do and I don't know that any of us are looking at that closely". She noted that it had not been a priority of testing agencies to address this "because we're working hard and fast; we still haven't done anything in particular to reach out to make sure we are representing different things well". She noted that OSCEs therefore "present, in general, a pretty narrow segment of patient problems and challenges to physicians". She added that she is very distant from education, and that, in general, the role of examination creation is now also distant from medical schools and medical education. The work that Danette McKinley has been doing at the ECFMG on race and gender concordance in examinee-standardized patient pairs described in the last chapter, is one of a very few working in the area that Smee identified as crucial. Yet, as many of the participants highlighted, there is a strong movement away from this research and toward the protection of data that legal considerations demand. Participants in large testing organizations expressed significant concerns that research will be more and more difficult to carry out in the future.

7.324 SPs versus Physicians as Raters

A second issue raised in the institutionalization of large exams is the role of "experts" in the testing process. All marking of live interactions in the US is now done by standardized patients (Whelan et al., 2005). This has long been a point of departure from Canadian OSCEs. According to Richard Reznick, who led creation of the Canadian national OSCE, in the US, "they had 16,000 people they had to test and they decided to create testing centres. I guess philosophically the big divide from the exam construction point-of-view was the use of SPs to score. Canadians continue to adopt the notion that if we're going to fail someone, a physician should be failing a physician, not a patient, not a standardized patient". Diana Tabak noted that the "American model" evolved because "they can't have clinicians observing as much as anybody would want, and therefore the responsibility has been imposed on standardized patients". Whelan said that when he was involved in OSCEs at the University of Southern California, students asked to have clinicians observing them. That is "students were not happy unless there were some guys in white coats there". Nevertheless, in the elaboration of the ECMFG and later NBME OSCEs, there would be no physician examiners present. Tabak thought this was inevitable because it is difficult to entice physicians to "give up their income to be involved in medical education". In addition, SPs are "a lot cheaper and a lot easier to control".

Richard Reznick noted that in developing the MCC OSCE "our business model included physicians giving their time [as] unpaid volunteers, given a small honorarium". He argued that the "hundreds and hundreds of physicians" who participate in the examination in Canada do so "in the spirit of an academic enterprise". Gerry Whelan at the ECFMG did point out that, although no physicians are present in OSCE stations, there is an assessment of the "clinical notes" written on every case in the ECMFG/NBME examination. These are later marked by physicians. Whelan explained that this was a compromise to deal with the absence of physician examiners. Although he cited for me a number of research studies relating to the validity of the clinical note, he added that it "was also a public relations thing having MDs help…. It was seen as a way to pacify people who felt we should be more like the Canadians".

In the UK, Harden addressed his view of using standardized patients to do marking by commenting that "it depends on what people are trying to achieve. I am not dismissing it as an approach and I can understand why the ECFMG would do this: it is one solution and it's better than no clinical exam. If it's either that or having no clinical exam and just MCQs, then that is infinitely better". However, he added that his "own view is, if possible, one should not go down that line" because "the public is expecting that [physicians] are going to judge". Tabak noted that a major constraint of this approach is that, "a standardized patient can't make clinical judgement and so they're given a tight script". It then becomes "checklist-driven to control [the] interaction". Harden argued that this model is "not really about educational theory or psychometrics, it's about the problem of logistics. If you are running an exam like the National Board all the time, then it's an expensive thing to do".

From the perspective of standardized patients, Robb argued that, "the biggest difference is that Canadians rightly insist on [physician] faculty observers as examiners. If I was taking a medical exam, I would want faculty observing me instead of a lay person who may have a limited understanding of how a checklist works". She went on to warn that if a candidate had reached a certain level of expertise, he or she "might fail the exam because they couldn't interpret it, if it wasn't on the 12 or 15 point checklist". She concluded, "I believe [in] an expert from the profession being the judge of whether a student is behaving or performing to the standards required".

When I questioned Robb about how this US-Canada difference arose, she called it "a big divide, a big shift in philosophy of how people are". When I probed about how the philosophical divide might be explained, she replied, "it is financial. When you take away a clinician's opportunity to earn income by being involved in these educational enterprises -- and the States is even more capitalistic than we are -- I think it's a financial decision". Tabak added to this that doctors are more resistant to being standardized than SPs. She observed that "sociologically, physicians are not standardizable". Thus, as production discourse takes hold with its focus on efficiency and standardization, one result has been the deprofessionalization of the physician role of examining. Seen in this light, some of the strong reactions elicited by the "American model" of SP-rated OSCE stations may be understood as resistance to the corporate proletarianization of the medical profession.[13]

Boulet, an ECFMG psychometrician, talked about the "wedge" issues arising from the cultural differences between the ECFMG and the NBME. He said that the reasons for the use of checklists in the national OSCE are "cost and resources". He also noted that the move away from requiring the presence of expert judges during examinations meant that long, detailed checklists have to be completed by standardized patients. In his view, "you are asking people to remember random points" because they do not have an expert ability to synthesize competent clinical performance. Validity suffers in that "you could get to the same point with only five or six key things" using what Boulet called "the jury method". In this model, a series of experts make global decisions about the competence of students taking the examination. He likened this to Olympic judges, arguing that expert judgment cannot effectively be broken down into detailed checklists administered by non-experts. Whelan noted that this discussion has now been lost, however, because the examination is in "production mode", and is no longer able to consider "holistic or global issues".

The shift to SP examiners led to the odd notion that "there are no evaluators in the room, there are merely observers". The implication is that the markers "are merely

---

[13] Magnusson (2000) has written about the link between the neo-liberal restructuring of higher education in North America and Taylorization of education. She cited the centrality of a Carnegie Foundation report called "Academic and Industrial Efficiency" (Cooke 1910), published by a disciple of Taylor, in achieving "the proletarianization of academic faculty".

identifying behaviours that individuals perform and [that] it is the responsibility of the test administrators to compile those records into evaluations and numbers". From this perspective, the "veracity" of the recording of the dispassionate and neutral observer is all that matters. One informant thought that research conducted from a "pure veracity perspective" illustrated that SPs "do a better, more accurate job". However, this person added that grading is not the neutral act of a dispassionate observer and that "OSCE scoring is highly interpretive act". These arguments clearly reflect a paradigm split about the function of the examiner in the room. I would contend, however, that there is something even more important going on. With the development of large-scale OSCE test centres, banks of cameras stream data to computers and unseen observers and, although SPs are grading candidates, they are doing so under scrutiny. They use measures created by and monitored by a whole host of observers. What is notable about examining in the production discourse is not who is in the room doing the examining, but who is outside the room watching. In fact, a huge number of unseen, anonymous observers who are not seen by the candidates at all, constitute a dramatic shift in the nature of surveillance in OSCEs.

In short, mounting a national OSCE for 25,000 US graduates per year rests on a particular "business model". This model of examination production relies on the use of standardized patients (at much lower cost) than the use of MD examiners. Once that model was adopted, the concept of expert physician raters was inadmissible. A routinized psychometric process of analysis (performed by people who some informants called "psychometric technicians") further led to rejecting the higher variability and uncertainty generated by global judgments. It was thus necessary to use "highly reliable" checklists.

Throughout my interviews at the ECFMG/NBME, the discourse of production was overt. One informant even termed the orientation to the examination "a manufacturing model", while another underscored that efficiencies of production were of paramount importance to the organization. Several used the industrial term "research and development" to refer to projects with names like the "NAV" - the "norming and validity study" and the "CAV" - the "collaboration and validity study". These were huge pilot studies, or in production discourse, "market tests" to judge the feasibility of the large-scale examination. I saw evidence of significant attention to "human resources", "finances" and "operations", just as one would find in any large industrial operation. One informant even noted that the Clinical Skills examination of the ECFMG/NBME is "both a brand and a model".

7.4   Thresholds and Resistances

During the 1990s and into the twenty-first century, OSCEs have appeared on a scale not seen before. These huge OSCEs require large amounts of money. Testing organizations such as the Medical Council of Canada, the National Board of Medical Examiners and the Education Commission of Foreign Medical Graduates Schools have developed "business plans" and have become more concerned with issues of finance and "economies of scale". Even medical schools moved from the small course-based OSCEs that were common in the 1970s and 1980s to larger, end-of-year OSCEs. A shift to production created opportunities but also constraints for standardized patients, psychometricians and health professionals who worked with OSCEs. A new level of administrators and trainers also emerged. Finally, while research continued, it concentrated on logistics and addressed the use of OSCEs in relation to health care labour needs, health care outcomes monitoring and international development.

The dominance of the production discourse means greater attention to accountability, in particular with regard to the "quality of the product"; to the uniformity of standards of professional work; and to the nature of professional labour. Negative side effects include the homogenization of examinations, reduced autonomy of teachers and schools, a reduced focus on formative assessment, and a shift from learning in medical schools to profit-driven examination preparation courses.

The development of the role of standardized trainers might be seen as a triumph for SPs. But the authority conferred along with this gendered position is limited. Though advancing in visibility in medical education, standardized patients have sought legitimacy in what is still an androcentric, medical and scientific environment. In contrast to the administrative and university positions available to those (mostly men) with psychometric and medical training, it is more difficult for standardized patients to access stable employment, good working conditions, institutional respect and career advancement. Their response has been to launch a professionalization project that uses professionalization discourse to define professional turf, inclusion and exclusion criteria, certification, and other classic features of professionalization and "closure" (Witz, 1992). Advancing their professionalization project will have major implications for OSCEs. First of all, it seems inevitable that there will be struggles for power within large testing organizations whose examinations depend on a constant supply of relatively cheap standardized patient labour. Defining competencies, standards of practice and fighting for autonomy will likely raise the economic aspirations of standardized patients, and they will find allies in the cohort of previous standardized patients who are now leaders in the same medical schools and testing organizations.

Second, a split is evident between those SPs involved in large scale examinations, and those who have skills and interest in teaching. Already, some tensions between the testing organizations that support the former and the universities that support the latter are apparent. Even Wallace, whose tone was decidedly positivist and progress-oriented, allows herself at the very end of her review to ever so gently question whether all of the developments in the standardized patient world that she has so carefully documented are in fact so positive. At the conclusion of her 22-page article, a lone paragraph intones her concerns about the massive shift in standardized patient work to examinations and assessment research, and away from teaching. She said, Standardized patient methodology is no longer in question. Yet, in our rush to quantify and establish its efficacy, a new question emerges. Have we not forgotten how much potential there is for standardized patients in other areas -- those wings on the caduceus? (Wallace, 1997, p. 25).

While the discourse of production is relatively new in relationship to the OSCE, there are already several areas of resistance visible.

7.41   Investing in Testing versus Teaching

There are limited resources for health professional education in all countries and large-scale examinations such as OSCEs are very expensive. While discussions of cost containment occupy those who mount large OSCEs, a less-discussed issue is

218

whether or not large-scale OSCEs can be cost-effective at all. Some argue that expensive methods of assessment divert money that might otherwise be available for teaching. Some suggest that while the large amounts of money invested in OSCEs may address issues such as accountability, they may actually impede good education. Ker in Dundee insists that "assessment is about how people learn, and how we can promote learning in our students". On the other hand, big examinations are about "practice issues, public accountability and the need to provide evidence". The cost of this, she suggests, is that "in having this big final exam instead of collecting evidence as you go along…people do all their work at the end, then get the assessment and think 'I can forget about it' -- that's not fostering reflection in our students at all". Boulet agreed, pointing out that the OSCE "works, but you do all this, you spend a ton of money, and the candidates pay to fail maybe 200 to 300 people a year [out of 25,000 tested] – and an eventual fail rate of zero. It's effective, but at what cost?" Similarly, Paula Stillman thought that OSCEs were "a very expensive model" for licensure and she added that "it's best used for formative feedback". Robb voiced similar points when she said "I think we are willing to pay more for testing because we need to be seen to be doing what is state of the art around the world. However, I'm not sure our tests are worth the money…. It is such a rich teaching tool that I would rather see the money go into a formative OSCE". Tabak said, after more than 25 years of working in both SP teaching and OSCEs, that "[I] have made up my mind" -- teaching is "where the resources should be".

On the day of our interview, Tabak had received a request over the listserv of the Association for Standardized Patient Educators asking for examples of "scripted answers" to be given to SPs in order to "ensure we are training our SPs appropriately in order to give exact answers on a high stakes OSCE". Tabak found this to be a very disturbing indication of the change in the role of SPs. As she saw it, "[w]e are caught up in summative OSCE and standardized things…and creating the exact same experience for every study so that it's fair, and you can't do that. You can't impose that kind of stricture on a relationship between a health professional and a patient". I recalled that she had started SP work in 1989, after a "horrible" experience with a physician, and has resolved to work to improve doctor-patient communication. I asked her to what extent she feels the creation of so many OSCEs has advanced that goal. Her response was, "I don't understand how that trains [better] health care professionals, I really don't". Similarly, one of the student informants said, "one of the flaws of the OSCE system is that you don't always get feedback and when you do it is way down the road and you don't remember". Boulet's response was consistent when he said, "I am not totally sold that the OSCE should be used for summative high stakes purposes. It was built to give rapid feedback for formative purposes".

Across the ocean in Scotland Sean McAleer agreed. He argued that "[u]nless you throw up on the dean's shoes or kill somebody, you're going to become a doctor". What then, is the value of constant and expensive summative assessment when it is not used to fail students? Ker told me that in shifting from smaller course-based OSCEs to larger school-wide OSCEs, "we are driven by logistics in delivering the OSCE because we've got 160 students that we have a morning to examine clinically. So the stations have to be four minutes. We have to run it in three sites. So it's like a military operation". If the value of the performance and the OSCE is learning and feedback, formative assessments would be much more appropriate, she concluded.

Two of the students I interviewed told me they had experienced many OSCEs during medical school and residency but had received feedback after none of them and Diana Tabak told me of a recent experience in which feedback was removed. She explained that the organizers found that the feedback "didn't jive with the assessment tool" and so they asked to remove it, telling her that feedback was "too costly and probably didn't mean anything anyway". By contrast, one of the students said in our interview, "the OSCEs in medical school, whether they are used to contribute to your mark at the end of the rotation or not, should be there so that you improve. It seems pointless to me to have an OSCE at the end… where you don't get feedback. Fully summative evaluation where you don't get any feedback at all… is at odds with calling it a school".

Paula Stillman, now director of a hospital, argued that with too much focus on "one final four-hour assessment", there is less emphasis on teaching with feedback and the development of skills at every step along the medical curriculum. As a result, she said, "in my role now in the hospital, [I see] very many physicians who have poor clinical skills. They rely on diagnostic studies to help them make diagnoses. They don't do histories and physicals and I think this is one of the reasons that the cost of medical care is so high. I think we have watered down clinical skills. I am not sure we have done the best job of teaching". She recounted a discussion she had with a teacher in Massachusetts about the cardiac exam. She recalled, "I was talking to her about having a student listen to the heart. She said, 'I can't do that either. Why should they listen when I can't do it? If I need something, I order an echo [cardiogram]'".

In the production model, one high-tech OSCE at the end of medical training may be like an expensive diagnostic test. Although designed to improve diagnosis, an over-reliance on such technology may, paradoxically, lead to deskilling physicians in the very areas of patient care that it is designed to improve.

7.42   Quality versus Cost Cutting and Efficiency

It is perhaps the contradiction between the mass production of scenarios and standardized patients necessary for the large scale OSCE that led Barrows to distance himself from their development. Although he was an early consultant for the National Board of Medical Examiners, Gliva-McConvey remembers attending an NBME meeting with him when he came out and dismissed the experience as "a test in a box". Gliva-McConvey was also concerned about the nature of this highly controlled examination that was so different than the simulated patient teaching cases that she had learned to create with Barrows. She was concerned that, "this was a national exam and everything had to be standardized and standardized. Patients are trained very, very strictly and there is not a lot of flexibility. There's not a lot of creativity, very set, very rigid, and that takes away from the creativity of an SP…" She added that, as a result, her SPs prefer not to work on NBME style OSCEs.

Sean McAleer similarly argued that "the very strength of the OSCE can be a weakness". In particular, he saw that "a lot of people hate being structured, having to do the same thing over and over again. There is no spontaneity. Their perception is that the role of the examiner disappears". In short, the experience of being part of an efficient machine is not appealing. Barrows also talked of his love for the unpredictability of performances and the fact that simulated patients can respond differently to different students; this flexibility make the process all the more effective. Further, Barrows argued, there should be a debriefing after every performance. As he put it, "I think the simulated patient should ask how they felt about it. What concerns they have, and then give them feedback on what they observed". But variability and feedback are not desirable characteristics in the production model.

A concern that was voiced by several key informants is the effect on quality of the constant search for efficiency. Anja Robb provided a critique of the compatibility of quality and efficiency in large-scale OSCEs. She argued that "most OSCE stations are put together too quickly, checklists are not field-tested, cases are not field-tested as much as they could be. I don't think checklists are as evidence-based as they could be. Some of the things being tested may not be best practices. I think a lot of busy, busy course directors, for the sake of expediency, will rely on stations that were acceptable 10 years ago, but are an embarrassment today.... I think that problem is because these people are suffering from the pressure of time". According to Robb, "somebody has to look at raising the bar in terms of how OSCEs are developed". She also argued that more collaboration is required between faculty members. The implication was that often the SP program is left to administer outdated materials, and that faculty do not have enough time to take an active role in examination creation and quality monitoring. Her point is that "quality suffers" when OSCE production is simply downloaded for implementation to the SP staff.

Barrows reflected on this issue and told me of his concerns that an exclusive focus on assessment moves away from the rich learning experience he created for his students 40 years ago. He was "concerned that the simulated patient was becoming mass-produced. And in becoming mass produced", Barrows worried about "quality control". He thought that in contrast with the "living, breathing" authenticity of early simulated patients, today authenticity is lost with the mass production of examinations. He attributed this partly to the presence of SP scripts and noted that his simulated patients never had scripts – just blank paper that they would fill in themselves. He said "I feel you get a wooden performance if they're trying to memorize how to behave. I love the spontaneous performance you get out of them".

In Dundee, Paul Preece, who ran the surgical OSCE for 20 years, expressed significant concern about the gradual reduction of station length from six minutes to five to four and a half and finally three and half minutes that was required as the number of students increased from 60 to 120 to 180. He called it "ridiculous" that the nature of assessment had fallen prey to "an efficiency criterion". Cohen also spoke about the rise of production discourse and her worry that the corporatization of OSCEs and SPs will lead to increasing ethical problems. She drew a parallel with what has happened in US in health care institution. As she put it, "I speak from an American perspective. If you took a historical perspective on the ideals behind HMOs [Health Management Organizations], at the beginning they were truly well intentioned. But [the movement] became very corrupted by corporations, by finance, by greed, by money". Cohen went on to say that in medical education, there are also "very strong, powerful bodies" and that because of "the way things sometimes flow in America" it seems to her essential that SPs must "speak out first, and become proactive" about what is important in training and what is important in feedback. She told me that, from her perspective, what happened in health care in America happened because "physicians didn't become proactive enough to do whatever they had to do to create a system that would work". She saw the rise of a corrupt system for which medicine is "paying a price. They've lost control over their own profession". For Cohen, the priority for SPs is the same: "not losing control over your own profession".

7.5 Summary

Production discourse began to have prominence in medical education generally, and testing particularly, in the 1990s. It is a dominant discourse today, particularly in North America. The language of production discourse comes from manufacturing and industry and its use has created new administrative and management roles in large-scale testing institutions. Throughout my interviews, I encountered frustration and resistance to this discourse. Participants pointed to the loss of focus on teaching and feedback; a move away from innovation and creativity; and a general degradation of human relations in the face of efficiency imperatives. These observations are familiar to those who have written about the effects of neo-liberal production discourses globally. In the words of Dhruvarajan, for example, "[t]he privileging of the economic aspects of life and the subordination of all other aspects, as the neo-liberal paradigm does, is seen as dehumanizing to all people, including those who gain financially (Dhruvarajan, 2005, p. 142).

CHAPTER 8: SURVEILLANCE: FROM VOYEURISM TO SELF-MONITORING

8.0   Introduction

This chapter summarizes my analysis of the three discourses elaborated in chapters five to seven -- performance, psychometrics and production -- and explores their inter-relationships. Then the implications of the dominance of this system of discourses for knowledge creation, for individuals and for institutional power are explored. Finally, I have speculated that the OSCE may once again undergo a transformation in the service of a new, emerging discourse constructing a trinity of technologies of self-monitoring.

8.1   OSCE Discourses and their Inter-Relations

The problem that now presents itself -- and which defines the task of a general history -- is to determine what form of relation may be legitimately described between these different series; what vertical system they are capable of forming; what interplay of correlation and dominance exists between them (Foucault, 1969/1972, p. 10).

In the last three chapters, I have sketched out the evidence that there are three discourses that make possible the object that is called OSCE. These are summarized in Table 7 below.

Table 7: Overview of the Three Discourses Related to OSCEs

Discourse	Miller's Pyramid and the Discourse of Performance	Cronbach's Alpha and the Discourse of Psychometrics	Taylorism and the Discourse of Production
Discursive statements	*Simulated patients and multi-station examinations (OSCEs) are tools for teachers to more fairly assess the performance of students and to provide feedback to students to enhance their skills*	*The OSCE is a measurement instrument for medical schools and testing organizations to reliably and validly assess the competence of candidates*	*The OSCE is a useful tool for assessment of competence for certification and licensure, and for public accountability because it is standardized, efficient and cost effective.*
Subject positions created by the discourse	Clinical teacher, inventor, patient instructor Simulated patient/model Student as performer	Psychometrician Standardized patient Student as candidate or data-point	Management Labour Student as raw material or product
Institutional locus of power	The medical classroom	The medical school, testing organizations	Institutions of testing, testing centres, regulatory bodies
Discursive concepts	Simulation and observation of performance	Reliability, validity and the conversion of human behaviour to numbers	Productivity and efficiency
Theoretical Choices	Behaviourism	Psychometrics	Production/Capitalism

Having elucidated these discourses in the previous chapters, it remains to "determine what form of relation may be legitimately described between these different series". As I have noted at several points in this research, the history of a discourse is studied by tracing its emergence, its points of dominance and the ebbs and flows of its explanatory power. It is important to underscore that the play of discourses I have presented is not unique to medicine. Certainly a sort of "origin" can be determined for each discourse, at least in so much as it is possible to locate moments when each first appeared in the medical literature or in the common parlance of educators. However, I should not like to imply that these moments of emergence were either fixed or unique. For example, the discourse of performance in medical education rose to prominence in the 1960s in association with the published works of Barrows and Harden. However, as I described in Chapter 5, the performance discourse was not *invented* in medical education. Rather it is a discourse that was imported from behaviourism, an epistemology dating to the early twentieth century and reflected in the work of Skinner (1953) and others. Psychometrics, by contrast, emerged in medical education in the 1980s, but was a well established discourse in psychology in America as early as the First World War (Hanson, 1993; Rose, 1985). Finally, while the production discourse emerged in medical education in the past decade, it did not arise *de novo* in medical education, but was imported from a much broader arena of economic activity associated with capitalism and neo-liberal globalization.

To explore the inter-relationships of the three discourses, I will first review briefly why they appeared in medical education in the places and at the times they did. Performance discourse was adopted in medical education in the 1960s at a time when institutions throughout North America and Europe were rocked by criticisms of oppressive hierarchy and rigid conservatism. Suspicions were expressed about traditional institutions. Calls for opening up of dialogue, of behaviour, of human rights and freedoms and of morals led to new ways of thinking about the purpose of educational institutions, of teachers, of students and of how and why knowledge is constructed. That medicine would re-examine and re-invent the nature of the teaching, of assessment and of the role of patients in medical education is therefore not surprising. Some of the inventive efforts to change the medical classroom, (such as the use of prostitutes and actors to teach) reflected fairly dramatic departures from traditional medical teaching. However, very quickly these changes shifted from teaching in the classroom to testing and examinations. The discourse of performance as a *method of assessment* had its roots less in the 1960s movement to address power differentials in the classroom (assessment itself being an act of power) and more in another discourse that rose to prominence in the 1960s -- that of science as a tool of social advancement and political control.

Movements such as "atoms for peace" tried to make a conceptual link between scientific methods and hope for "a better world" (Eisenhower, 1953). The space race of the 1960s pitted major world powers against one another in an attempt to exert dominance over each other via scientific discovery. Medicine, steeped in science since the eighteenth century, expanded the targets at which scientific method could be aimed. The emergence of performance discourse reflected the recognition that what were once considered "soft" aspects of medical practice -- the doctor patient relationship, empathy, communication skills -- could be given the same attention as the "harder" elements of medical scientific knowledge. Attention meant testing, and a frenzy of performance-based methods arose. Medicine already had at its disposal a powerful epistemology to use in moving toward the assessment of performance. What Foucault characterized as the "medical gaze" (Foucault, 1963/2003), the penetrating observation that allowed doctors to classify and to "know" patients, needed simply to be redirected to students. Hunter argued, the school is, in fact, purposely created for such functions.

[T]he detailed organization of the school as a purpose-built pedagogical environment is assembled from a mix of physical and moral elements: special architectures; devices for organizing space and time; body techniques; practices of surveillance and supervision; pedagogical relationships; procedures of administration and examination (Hunter, 1996, p. 147).

The creation of simulated patients and then of multi-station OSCEs therefore was a logical development in the quest for "scientific technologies" that could bring what were previously only loosely controlled elements of physician performance under surveillance and control within medical schools.

The psychometric discourse, where it took hold, did not replace this performance discourse so much as it transformed it. In the 1980s, there were seismic shifts in the west as the social-democratic systems that had created the welfare states of post World War II began to be replaced by neo-liberal governments keen to reconfigure systems of education and healthcare by transferring management to private sector organizations and companies (Teeple, 2000). This shift was accompanied by a discourse of accountability that required measurement (Dowdle, 2006). Medical education and medical schools were not left out of these changes and, in the United States in particular, health services and educational institutions were privatized, or were required to implement measures of outcome and performance. Thus it is not a surprise that during this period, medical education discovered the science of psychometrics, a technology that propelled the rising profession of psychology earlier in the twentieth century (Gould, 1981; Rose, 1985) and a field that had been associated with the military since the Second World War (Hanson, 1993). European countries, which retained social-welfare systems to a larger degree than the United States, gave somewhat less credence to models of psychometric measurement (Canada was intermediate) resulting in the very different prominence of psychometric discourse today on the two sides of the Atlantic. A more recent implication of this differential adoption of psychometric discourse is the more obvious criticism of psychometric models of assessment being published by European medical educators (e.g. Schurwirth & van der Vleuten, 2005).

Where it is dominant, it can be argued that psychometric discourse paved the way for the emergence of a discourse of production. Psychometricians originally aimed for standardization and reduction of statistical variance in the analysis of performance. But it was a small leap to the standardization of everything related to testing, including the roles of employees, the design of testing centres and the behaviour of students. This small leap was medical education's adoption of principles of manufacturing. By the late 1990s, neo-liberal reorganization of all institutions in North America was well underway, prioritizing the movement of goods and services within and between countries, the reduction of costs and the efficiency of production (Teeple, 2000). As Magnusson has argued, this also led to a restructuring of higher education curricula, pedagogical methods, governance and administration in order to support neo-liberal ideology and objectives (Magnusson 2000). Whereas national governments have been adopting outsourcing of patient care as a means of reducing cost (sending patients to other countries where medical treatments are less expensive) since the 1990s, new programs are now developing with the goal of creating similarly mechanisms to globalize medical education, including the development of "international standards" and "globalized examinations" (Segouin, Hodges & Brechat, 2005). Efforts are aimed at facilitating an increasingly mobile medical labour force. But as Battiste has argued, "claiming universality often means aspiring to domination. Universality underpins cultural and cognitive imperialism, which establishes a dominant group's knowledge, experience, culture and language as the universal norm" (Battiste, 2005, p. 124).

Expansion and domination are increasingly common themes in the universalization of America-centric models of medical education, including the establishment of western medical schools and examination models in countries where "production costs" are lower (Segouin et al., 2005). Inevitably, such efforts to bring medical education, assessment and licensure into the domain of manufacturing have created large and powerful, globalizing testing institutions. In the words of Torfing, "the largest Fordist factories were constructed as exemplary models for the design of both public and private institutions" (Torfing, 1999, p. 229).

8.2   Shifts in the Play of Power: From Seduction to Pornography

The development of testing is an outstanding example of Foucault's thesis that power has been evolving in the direction of increasing efficiency, subtlety and scope. Especially remarkable is that people have increasingly found themselves in the position where they feel their only recourse is to ask, even to insist, that they undergo the pornographic scrutiny of tests. Power has become refined indeed when people demand that they be subjected to it (Hanson, 1993, p. 306).

Looking at the OSCE as I have above, it is possible to see the plays of power at institutional, governmental and societal levels. First, the development of technologies of observation led to the invention of simulations and OSCEs. Later, as psychometric imperatives swept through medical education, statistically derived concepts of reliability and validity created power for those individuals and institution with this particular expertise. Finally and most recently, adoption of production discourse in a context of globalization is creating powerful institutions that look more like factories than schools.

But if the lens is turned around to examine the particular implications of these discourses for *individuals* (Smith's (2004) "local practices of discourse"), what we see is equally compelling. I would argue that the discourse of performance created a triadic model of surveillance as shown in Figure 5. Originally, a powerful male physician observed while a medical student examined a passive female model (simulated patient). With the rise of the psychometric discourse however, there was a shift, as depicted in Figure 6. The patient -- re-baptized a "standardized patient" -- became a standardized "tool", trained carefully to present a role created by an invisible set of authors who were medically, but increasingly also psychometrically-oriented. She was also now an *observer*. However her observations were not entirely her own; she recorded them on standardized checklists given to her by trainers. A physician was present in most cases to ensure that everything took place in a desired fashion and to assess elements that the standardized patient could not. Thus, the shift from a discourse of performance to a discourse of psychometrics changed the nature of surveillance. No longer were all of the players in the room. Significant power was shifted outside the room and outside of the primary student interactions to unseen observers. An element of *anonymity* of power was built into the process of surveillance, which was *extra-local*[14].

These relationships became even more complex with the emergence of the production discourse, as shown in Figure 7. While only fully realized in the United States in institutions such as the new National Board of Medical Examiners testing centres, elements of this new set of relationships can be seen in production-oriented OSCEs around the world. In the full blown production model, there are only *two* people physically present in an OSCE station. The student interacts with the standardized patient who records his or her every utterance and gesture on pre-prepared checklists and ratings. No physician is actually present in the room, and often not even at the examination. Instead, two to three cameras record all interactions and send a constant stream of data to banks of powerful computers. Where standardized information

---

[14] The term "extra-local" was introduced by Dorothy Smith (Campbell 2003).

management systems cannot be assumed to produce 'quality' assessments, physicians review, at a later time and in a separate location, videos or notes generated during the examination. Physician examiners are thus completely disembodied from the examination process. The triad of the original performance discourse is thus replaced by a whole hierarchy of anonymous, extra-local observers including physicians, psychometricians and managers who watch in real or asynchronous time from *outside* the station. This fundamental shift in the nature of the technology is captured in the three schematics below.

Figure 5: An OSCE Station Arising from the Discourse of Performance

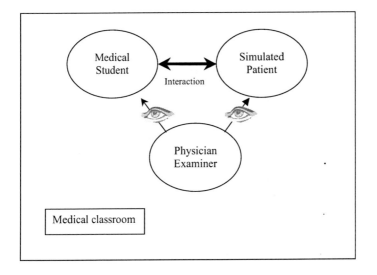

Figure 6: An OSCE Station Arising from the Discourse of Psychometrics

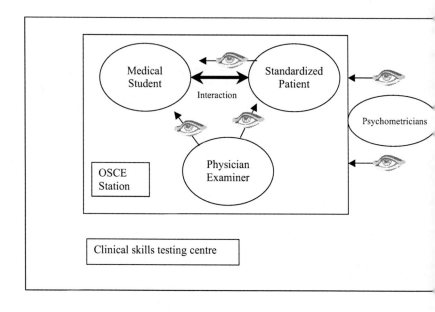

Figure 7: An OSCE Station Arising from the Discourse of Production

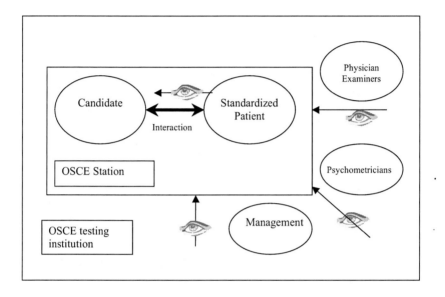

The graphic representations in Figures 5 to 7 illustrate how the different discourses have created dramatically different experiences for students but also for those who surround them and observe them in the process of testing.

Several features are apparent. First, with the addition of a psychometric lens, the external, or extra-local, surveillance became more formalized. Certainly a physician examiner sitting in the room always brought with him/her the "normalizing gaze" and judgement of the medical profession. Within a psychometric discourse, however, the physician too came under surveillance for the first time. Further, in the change from simulated patients to standardized patients, the woman in the room was no longer simply a "model" or "tool", but now had a dual role that involved both performance and the reporting of data to those outside of the room. These shifts were taken much further with the production model in which no physician examiner is in the room at all. Video and audio technologies convey sound and images to a multiplicity of silent observers. Observation is thus completely anonymized and displaced. The "candidate" cannot see the faces of his or her observers. The standardized patient must be treated like a patient, even while the student knows that she is also observing and assessing.

If Foucault's work on the medical gaze helps us to understand why medicine moved to observing students directly in the 1960s, his work on the panopticon clarifies these technological mutations of OSCEs. Foucault argued that the design of schools, hospitals and prisons in the last two centuries has made possible a generalized surveillance of individuals. He used Bentham's "Panopticon", a circular building in which the occupant of every room (or cell) could be seen from a centre observation point, as a structural metaphor for the ideal architecture of surveillance (Foucault, 1975/1995). In a chapter called *The Means of Correct Training,* Foucault outlined two fundamental disciplining procedures brought into play with the architecture of the panopticon: "hierarchical observation" and "normalizing judgment" He wrote,
The examination combines the techniques of an observing hierarchy and those of a normalizing judgment. It is a normalizing gaze, a surveillance that makes it possible to qualify, to classify and to punish. It establishes over individuals a visibility though which one differentiates and judges them (Foucault, 1975/1995, p. 184-5).

236

OSCEs have become machines of both hierarchical judgment and a normalizing gaze; the refinement of which has increased as the technology moved through discourses of performance to psychometrics to production.

Hierarchical observation includes four technologies, according to Foucault. The first technology is the placement of individuals in enclosures that are partitioned into rooms where each performs his or her functions. Supervision is facilitated by an architecture that creates a cellular structure: cells in prisons, workstations in factories, classrooms in schools and "stations" in OSCEs. Based on the model of a military camp, the highly structured and partitioned spaces of modern buildings enclose, control and supervise individuals and regulate their behaviours. An OSCE test centre, with its rows of identical rooms, streaming digital images to a central control room, is designed to allow observers to "know, control and alter" those inside. Like the military camp, the prison or the school building, surveillance and control of behaviour is facilitated because one gaze sees everything constantly.

The second technology linked to hierarchical observation, according to Foucault, is control of activity according to time -- the most efficient means being a "timetable". Assigning strict units of time to govern the activities of individuals in all aspects of life controls the workplace and the classroom. Similarly, OSCEs use "rotation schedules" with strictly regulated time intervals to ensure that each encounter is measured and allocated the same interval of time. Movements are controlled by stop watches and buzzers.

The third technology involves concluding each segment of performance with an evaluative judgment. Report cards, case histories, prison dossiers and performance appraisals are familiar forms of such judgment. In OSCEs, judgment is even more extensive as behaviours in each and every station are observed and documented using a complex set of "checklists" and "ratings".

Finally, Foucault's fourth technology linked to hierarchical observation is to embed within the process of observation a system of differentiation such that each individual is classified according to a set of defining characteristics. Schools, hospitals, prisons and all other modern institutions have categories in which all individuals are classified, ranked or rated in order to triage their individual futures. In OSCEs, assigning scores for various sub-domains of performance allows participants to be classified, determining their future possibilities. The ultimate goal of hierarchical observation, said Foucault, is the "increasing, linear perfection of each individual according to a social design" (Foucault, 1975/1995, p. 186).

All of these disciplinary measures are part of "normalizing judgment", a process that operates in disciplinary systems through codes that punish certain behaviours and reward others. All aspects of disciplinary function are controlled by reference to such codes, which in OSCEs are expressed as "competencies". "Competencies", in turn, dictate which professional behaviours are appropriate, and which are not, as operationalized by rating scales. Thus we can trace the line of professional power from the grading of examinations directly to behavioural normalization, via the intermediary of behavioural checklists and rating forms.

Hanson wrote about the shift in examination technology from the use of interactions in which the student tries to "persuade" another person (teacher, supervisor or mentor) that he or she is competent, to the use of "voyeuristic surveillance" in which examiners are not physically present but instead gaze from behind metaphorical or real one-way mirrors. He argued that the construction of social relations, when all players are present in the room, is characterized by efforts of the student being assessed to present the him or herself in a convincing and competent way (as described by Goffman, 1959). He likened this kind of performance to "seduction". This dynamic operates in the triadic OSCE station that is constructed by performance discourse, as depicted in Figure 5. However said Hanson, removing observers to extra-local positions drastically changes the dynamic. He said,
If the artful presentation of Goffman's self is seductive, what happens in testing is, to borrow a simile from Jean Baudrillard, pornographic. Pornography differs from seduction in that the individual fixed by the pornographic gaze is powerless to conceal, control, or nuance anything. She or he is displayed for the observer's inspection, recreation, probing, and penetration in whatever way satisfies his or her purely selfish purposes (Hanson, 1993, pp. 304-306).

To extend Hanson's metaphor, the OSCE constructed by production discourse, as depicted in Figure 7, is a peep-show.

In summary then, OSCEs function as technology at two levels. At the level of what Smith (2004) calls the "local practices of discourse", OSCEs shape and alter the possibilities for individuals through surveillance and hierarchical observation. At the macro-sociological level, OSCEs function as production-oriented technologies, adaptable to the economic imperatives of efficiency and standardization. This combination of hierarchical control and scientific management characterize and propel current political-economic discourse (Torfing, 1999). In other word, OSCEs are much more than simple innovations for the assessment of students, they are powerful instruments of "governmentality" in the Foucauldian (1979/1991) sense. [15] Seen this way, OSCEs are elements of a "decentred process" of control and is "decomposed into political rationalities, governmental programs, technologies and techniques of government" (O'Malley, Weir and Shearing, 1997, p. 501).

8.3   Power, Testing and the Future of the OSCE in Medicine

In this research, I have studied in detail how the technology called the OSCE is part of different discourses that define what is "seeable and sayable". What is "thinkable" is also made possible by these discourses. I have also shown that what an OSCE *is*, varies in time and in place according to the discursive elements -- statements, enunciative modalities and concepts - that make it possible in diverse forms.

An obvious conclusion arising from this research is that the OSCE will continue to evolve as discourses change and as emergent ones make possible different statements, objects, subject positions and institutions. I am, therefore, curious about what might emerge next. In fact, I have been alert to words and ideas that might signal the next discursive irruption. If I might look into the future in a way that is based more on conjecture than evidence, I could draw together a set of words and ideas that is appearing more and more often in medical education and that includes: "reflection, self-directed learning, insight" and the beginning of calls for "learning contracts,

---

[15] O'Malley, Weir and Shearing synthesis Foucault's notion of governmentality as "the nexus between political rationalities and the technologies of rule" (1997, p. 503).

portfolios and self-directed assessment". Nelson and Purkis (2004) have argued that "mandatory reflection" is a powerful emerging discourse in the health professions. While I had not initially found any systematic links between a discourse of reflection and the OSCE *per se*, I did notice the emergence of this discourse in medical education assessment more generally. For example, the Canadian Royal College of Physicians and Surgeons has begun to require the submission of self-directed, reflective learning diaries as evidence of maintenance of competence (RCPSC 2006). This led me to speculate (Hodges, 2004) that a discursive "trinity" of the technologies (self-reflection, self-assessment and self-regulation) similar to what Foucault described in his work on ethics and governmentality (Foucault, 1997), may be emerging in medical education.

Foucault (1997) believed that the use of power in liberal democracies was shifting to rely less and less on overt displays of state power. Instead, governance, he said, was increasingly accomplished through a host of disseminated and dispersed technologies. He argued that professional disciplines are particularly effective means of controlling behaviour at a considerable distance from state governments. Not only are professional disciplines central to surveillance and governmental control of their members, he said, but the methods by which they do so are increasingly subtle and more distributed. They achieve their greatest power when those acted upon administer technologies of control upon themselves (Foucault, 1972-1977/1980). Rose showed how distributed strategies of surveillance and governance are dependent upon institutions (schools, the domesticated family, the lunatic asylum, the prison) that promise to create individuals who do not need to be governed by others, but who will govern themselves, master themselves, care for themselves (Rose, 1996, p. 45).

Given these arguments, it seems only a matter of time until the technologies of self-reflection, self-assessment and self-regulation come to reshape the OSCE once again and make it a useful tool for the transformation of individuals through internalized "technologies of the self". Usher and Edwards have suggested that individuals are increasingly placing themselves under their own surveillance and that, in the future, will control themselves, not through "external" discipline, but by applying disciplinary techniques of confession and self-examination (Usher & Edwards, 1994, pp. 50-51).

It is possible that the ever-malleable OSCE will not be able to accommodate this shift; the change from an external to an internal locus of surveillance may not be possible with its technologies. It may also simply collapse under the weight of its great financial demands. On the other hand, the OSCE has proved to be a highly resilient technology, adapted effectively for knowledge creation and for channelling of power across three very different discourses. Can it be once again modified to serve the trinity of self-reflection, self-assessment and self-regulation?

Hanson said,

If one were to imagine the next step in the perfection of power by testing, it would be for people to *request* that they be tested in circumstances of general suspicion, as they already ask to be tested when they are under individualized suspicion. At first glance, such a development seems preposterous. Why would anyone demand a test to prove that they are not doing something that nobody accuses or specifically suspects them of doing in the first place? To bring this about would mark a truly ingenious extension of power (Hanson, 1993 p. 306).

Wondering about the fusion of "self-monitoring" and the "OSCE", I searched for these terms in the medical education literature. Only one paper appeared, but what it said made me sit bolt upright:

Final-year residents in Obstetrics and Gynaecology at the University of Toronto created OSCE stations in preparation for their certification examination. Residents were asked to compare resident-created stations with faculty-created stations. The students found every aspect of OSCE development to be of educational benefit. Residents perceived the benefits of the OSCE sessions to be greater than equivalent lengths of time spent in traditional group study sessions. CONCLUSIONS: A self-directed learning approach, based on OSCE development and implementation, shows promise as a learning aid at the senior residency level. We suggest a controlled trial designed to objectively measure outcomes of this learner-centred approach (Windram, Thomas, Rittenberg, Bodley, Allan & Byrne, 2004, p. 815).

CHAPTER 9: REFLECTIONS

It was difficult, at the outset of my research, to imagine what sort of contribution I might make. In reflecting on my experience now, I believe there are a number of possible implications, both at a public level and at a personal level. First, I have created what I believe to be the first socio-history of performance based assessment in general, and of the OSCE in particular. The research I have undertaken is both methodologically and epistemology distinct from what has been written before. I hope that this might be of interest to other researchers, educators and those involved in examinations. Second, there are very few research studies of any kind in medical education that use Foucauldian methodology. I hope that I have been sufficiently explicit about the development of a method of discourse analysis that other researchers could draw on my work for future studies. Third, I think I have sounded a warning bell about the excesses of the emerging production discourse and its link to academic capitalism. The move to production has been accompanied by a degradation of education (no student feedback); impoverishment of human relations (extra-local surveillance in place of face-to-face interaction); inappropriate reliance on simulation (simulation doctors who learn "fake empathy"); removal of actual patients in education; reduction of choice of educational methods and technologies (monopolization); narrowing of the diversity of cases and patients (through standardization); and threats to equity (marginalization of women and minorities both in 'ghettos' of part-time OSCE work).

There are also important implications for me personally. I began this thesis by citing Jana Sawicki's writing about the place of reflection in Foucauldian research. She argued,

One's commitment to poststructuralist methods and analysis must itself always be subject to reappraisal.... One of the redeeming features of Foucault's discourse for me has been its continual resistance to efforts to turn it into a political orthodoxy. Foucault's discourse invites its own critique. Moreover, the shifts in the trajectory of his research were evidence of his willingness to surpass himself (Sawicki, 1991, p. 7).

Thinking about the idea of trying to surpass oneself, I re-examined my own previous academic writing which, to a large extent, reflected the discourses I have written

242

about here at such length. Of course, when I was writing my earlier papers, I did not think in terms of discourse, nor did I recognize the paradigms to which the words I chose were tied. I did not start my academic career until the early 1990s, by which time the performance discourse was well established. In one of my earliest papers, I discussed how the OSCE might be brought
to my own field of psychiatry, and used mostly performance discourse, but also some rudimentary psychometric arguments (Hodges & Lofchy, 1997) to support this contention. During the next five years I became Director of Undergraduate Education for the University of Toronto, Department of Psychiatry and while I oversaw all examinations, I published a series of articles on OSCEs and reliability (Hodges, Regehr, Hanson & McNaughton, 1997), validity (Hodges, Regehr, Hanson & McNaughton, 1998), the properties of measurement instruments (Hodges, Regehr, McNaughton, Tiberius & Hanson, 1999; 2002). I also collaborated with a number of colleagues publishing articles on OSCEs and simulation in family medicine, internal medicine, surgery and communication skills training (e.g. Hodges, Turnbull, Cohen, Bienenstock & Norman, 1996). It was during this period that I completed my masters of education at the Ontario Institute for Studies in Education where I learned much of the methodology and literature that I utilized in these works. I studied with professors who were publishing from a psychometric perspective. The master's program exposed me to a broader perspective on education, including the different histories and roles of the university and of professions. I also caught some glimpses of issues of power related to the medical profession.

After 1998, I was increasingly involved with national and international education and testing organizations, including serving on the OSCE test committee for the Medical Council of Canada. I became Director of Examinations for the Ontario International Medical Graduate Program. This led to a shift and the articles I wrote or co-authored more often addressed the implementation of larger scale OSCEs in Canada (Hodges & Herold-McIlroy, 2003), the UK (Sauer, Hodges, Santhouse & Blackwood, 2005) and China (Stern, Friedman Ben-David, De Champlain, Hodges, Wojtczak & Schwarz, 2005). I recognize in these articles the institutional production discourse identified in this research. During this time, I was not involved in formal education or exposed to critical theoretical work. This changed in 2001 when I enrolled in the PhD program at the Ontario Institute for Studies in Education, with a goal of deepening my understanding of theory in relation to assessment. Through a set of courses that was much theoretically richer than those I had taken during my master's program, I encountered ideas about equity, academic capitalism, post-structuralism, discourse and other schools of thought.

The transformative effect on my thinking and on my research is evident in this thesis, but also in some of my newer publications. In the last few years, I have published a sociologic analysis of the constructive nature of simulation (Hodges, 2003a), a critique of the psychometric concept of validity (Hodges, 2003b), a discussion of Foucault's notion of subjectivity and the medical gaze in assessment (Hodges, 2004) and a historiography of alternate perspectives in the history of medical education (Hodges, 2005). I passed through a fairly long psychometric phase; then used an institutional production discourse; and most recently have begun to adopt a critical, constructivist perspective on assessment and OSCEs.

Muzzin has expressed the difficulties she experienced in taking a critical perspective while being within a health professional faculty. Writing about academic capitalism and its repressive effects on equity in pharmacy, she wrote, "I had a lot of trouble even coming to the point of being able to reflect on the problem" (Muzzin, 2005, p. 149). Similarly, I recognize a rather long trajectory in my career from the realization that there were negative effects of examinations in general, to seeing the degree to which they were part of an interlocking system of discourse that was creating and constructing these negative effects in my own environment. Further, I see now more clearly, although not completely, some of the ways in which the perspectives and roles I have taken on are "embedded in the very same discourses and practices of power that 'my' research sought to understand" (Delhi, 2003, p. 140). Although pleased about this transformation, I am aware that Delhi has sounded a caution about "accounts of the 'constituent subject' who stands on the side of freedom in opposition to power, who speaks truth in response to ideology". Her worry is that this leads to the researcher to believe that they can "assist the long silenced and alienated others to be 'restored' to themselves, to provide a space where those who are marginalized can 'come to voice'" (Dehli, 2003, p. 141). Rather, she wrote,

Foucault's genealogical investigations recommended suspicion in relation to such accounts, not because he believed that control, domination, and violence have become irrelevant, but because *modern* power operates across many different registers, through different networks, and though direct and indirect 'productive' means. In particular, his investigations asked about the ways in which forms and practices of knowledge operate to produce particular kinds of subjects as their effect (Dehli, 2003, p. 141).

With my new-found perspective on knowledge production and power in relation to OSCEs, how then might I proceed? Post-structuralist research is sometimes criticized as being idealist, and not placing sufficient emphasis on action. Sawicki argued, however, that Foucauldian research can be adapted for action and that while a Foucauldian analysis alone does not constitute a *plan* for action; it does create an analysis of power and knowledge production that can be helpful for taking concrete steps to counteract the negative effects of the flow of power. She wrote,

Foucault's theories do not tell us what to do, but rather how some of our ways of thinking and doing are historically linked to particular forms of power and social control. His theories serve less to explain than to criticize and raise questions. His histories of theory are designed to reveal their contingency and thereby free us from them (Sawicki, 1991, p. 47).

It is the "freeing" effect that I have experienced most powerfully by undertaking this research. Seeing the practices around me, and those in which I engage myself, as constructions that arise as part of the reproduction of different discourses has opened up the possibility of choices that I had not recognized previously. Publicly articulating the idea that OSCEs, SPs and even medical education in general are constructed in various ways, at various times because of different discourses, has been a new insight for some of the individuals who have spoken to me after I have presented these ideas at recent conferences. If practices, roles and institutions arise because of certain discourses, then presumably it might be possible to tackle some of the inequities and distortions in education by trying to dislodge or delegitimize problematic discourses. Hanson wrote that,

[T]ests are instruments of the evolving system of dominating institutions that act to curtail individual freedom and dignity. Therefore, it is almost inevitable for a study that seeks to explore the human consequences of testing to include a critique and some proposals for how its more destructive effects might be restrained (Hanson,

1993, p. 7).

The ways to address the more destructive effects of examinations are not fully obvious to me at this juncture, but the desire to identify them will serve to guide the next stages of my work. I hope to explore how concepts of ethics and equity might be brought to bear on discourses about assessment and examination. Even now I see the outline of an approach in the writings of those who critique the state of society more generally. As Dhruvarajan has written, "[t]he goal is to promote conditions for the adaptation of diverse ways of life including diverse economic paradigms. The crucial point is to recognize that people should be free to choose a particular way of life that is in keeping with their history and culture. They should be free to choose appropriate terms of trade, appropriate technology, and an appropriate form of government that works best for them" (Dhruvarajan, 2005, p. 139). Magnusson points out that, despite the dominance of hegemonic neo-liberal discourses, there are "important and emancipatory movements in areas such as health, environment, social equity and democracy" and that one can work toward "increased vigilance" in terms of "redirecting the activities organized through post-secondary education toward cultural work that is consistent with the various emancipatory efforts" (Magnusson, 2000, p. 123).

Working to find ways to re-introduce choice and freedom into what Foucault called our "examined society" is a worthy occupation in a community of scholars. The completion of this analysis, which exposes the excesses of what Foucault would have called our current "regimes of truth", is a first step in my participation in that community.

CHAPTER 10: BIBLIOGRAPHY

Abrahamson, S. (1985). The oral examination: The case for and against. In J. S. Lloyd & D. G. Langley (Eds.), *Evaluating the skills of medical specialists.* (pp. 121-124). Chicago: American Board of Medical Specialties.

Abrahamowicz, M., Tamblyn, R. M., Ramsey, J. O., Klass, D. K., & Kopelow, M. (1990). Detecting and correcting for rater-induced differences in standardized patient tests of clinical competence. *Academic Medicine*, 65(9), S25-26.

Adamo, G. (2003). Simulated and standardized patients in OSCE: achievements and challenges 1992-2003. *Medical Teacher*, 25(3), 262-270.

Ainsworth, M. A., Rogers, L. P., Markus, J. F., Dorsey, M. D., Blackwell, T. A., & Petrusa, E. R. (1991). Standardized patient encounters: A method for teaching and evaluation. *Journal of the American Medical Association*, 266(10), 1390-1396.

Albert, M., Hodges, B., Lingard, L., & Regehr, G. (2006). La recherché en éducation médicale: entre le service et la science. *Pédagogie Médicale*, (In Press).

Anderson, W.A., & Harris, I.B. (2003). Arthur S. Elstein, Ph.D.: Skeptic, scholar, teacher and mentor. *Adv Health Sci Educ Theory Pract.* 8(2):173-82.

Anderson, M. B., Stillman, P. L., & Wang, Y. (1994). Growing use of standardized patients in teaching and evaluation in medical education. *Teaching and Learning in Medicine*, 6(1), 15-22.

Andrew, R., & Bates, J. (2000). Program for licensure for international medical graduates in British Columbia: 7 years' experience. *Canadian Medical Association Journal, 162*(6), 801-803.

Bakhtin, M. M. (1981). *The dialogic imagination: Four essays by M. M. Bakhtin* (C. Emerson and M. Holquist, Trans.) Austin: University of Texas Press.

Bark H, & Cohen R. (2002). Use of an objective, structured clinical examination as a component of the final-year examination in small animal internal medicine and surgery. *Journal of the American Veterinary Medical Association, 221*(9), 1262-1265.

Barrows, H. S., & Abrahamson, S. (1964). The programmed patient: A technique for appraising student performance in clinical neurology. *Journal of Medical Education, 39*, 802-805.

Barrows, H. S. (1971). *Simulated patients (Programmed patients): The development and use of a new technique in medical education.* Springfield, Ill: Charles C Thomas Publishers.

Barrows H. S. (1993). An overview of the uses of standardized patients for teaching and evaluating clinical skills. *Academic Medicine*, 68(6), 443-451.

Battiste M. (2005). You can't be the global doctor if you're the colonial disease. In P. Tripp & L. Muzzin (Eds.), *Teaching as activism: Equity meets environmentalism* (pp. 121-133). Montreal & Kingston: McGill-Queen's University Press.

Beck, J. B. (1966). *Medicine in the American colonies*. New York: Horn and Wallace Publishers. (Originally published in 1850).

Becker, H., Geer, B., Hughes, E., & Strauss, A. (1961). *Boys in White*. Chicago: University of Chicago Press.

Becker, F. & Steele, F. (1995). *Workplace by design: Mapping the high-performance workscape*. San Francisco, CA: Jossey-Bass Publishers.

Becker, H.S., Geer, B., & Hughes, E.C. (1968). *Making the grade: The academic side of college life*. New York: John Wiley and Sons, Inc.

Bell, M. (2006). *Patient Partner Program*. Retrieved May 17, 2006, from http://www.arthritis.ca/programs%20and%20resources/patientpartners/default.asp?s=1.

Ben-David, M. F., Klass, D. J., Boulet, J., De Champlain, A., King, A. M., Pohl, H. S. et al. (1999). The performance of foreign medical graduates on the National Board of Medical Examiners (NBME) standardized patient examination prototype: a collaborative study of the NBME and the Educational Commission for Foreign Medical Graduates (ECFMG). *Medical Education*, 33(6), 439-446.

Bernstein B. (1990). *Class, codes and control: The structuring of pedagogic discourse (Vol. 4)*. London: Routledge.

Billings, J. A., & Stoeckle, J.D. (1977). Pelvic examination instruction and the doctor-patient relationship. *Journal Medical Education*, 52(10), 834-839.

Bonner, T. N. (1995). *Becoming a physician: Medical education in Britain, France, Germany and the United States, 1750-1945*. New York: Oxford University Press.

Brailovsky, C. A., Grand'Maison, P., & Lescop, J. (1992). A large-scale, multi-centre Objective Structured Clinical Examination for licensure. *Academic Medicine, 67*(10), S37-39.

Brennan R. L. (1983). *Elements of generalizability theory*. Iowa City, Iowa: American College Testing Program.

Brennan, R. L. (1997). A perspective on the history of generalizability theory. *Educational Measurement: Issues and Practice, 16*(4), 14-20.

Broadbent, J. & Laughlin, R. (1997) In Broadbent, J. (Ed.) *The end of the professions?* London: Routledge.

Brown, R. E. (1979). *Rockefeller medicine men: Medicine and capitalism in America*. Berkeley, California: University of California Press.

Burgess, J. H., & Hurteau, G. D. (2004). Our new Royal College headquarters: The road to the monastery. In H. B. Dinsdale & G. Hurteau (Eds.), (pp. 33-47). *The evolution of specialty medicine: 1979-2004*. Ottawa: Royal College of Physicians and Surgeons of Canada.

Campbell, M. (2003). Dorothy Smith and knowing the world we live in. *Journal of Sociology and Social Welfare*, 30(1):

Canadian Cancer Society, National Cancer Institute of Canada, Lederle Laboratories, & Associated Medical Services. (1992). *Consensus Statement on the teaching and assessment of communication skills in Canadian medical schools*. Toronto: Canadian Cancer Society.

Canguilhem, G. (1980). What is psychology? (H. Davis, Trans.) *Ideology and Consciousness,* 7, 37-50 (Original work published in 1956).

Carpenter, J. (1995). Cost analysis of Objective Structured Clinical Examinations. *Academic Medicine, 70*(9), 828-833.

Clark, G. A. (2000). *Objective structured clinical examination (OSCE): An easier way forward.* Unpublished thesis. Diploma in Management Studies, Dundee Graduate School of Management, University of Albertay. Dundee, Scotland.

Coburn D. (1993). Professional power in decline: Medicine in a changing Canada. In F. W. Hafferty & J. B. McKinlay (Eds.), *The changing medical profession: An international perspective* (pp. 92-103). New York: Oxford University Press.

College of Family Physicians of Canada (2006). *College of Family Physicians of Canada.* Retrieved April 28, 2006, from http://www.cfpc.ca/.

College of Massage Therapists of Ontario (2005). *College of Massage Therapists of Ontario.* Retrieved September 30, 2005, from http://www.cmto.com/index.html.

Colliver, J. A., Vu, N. V., Marcy, M. L., Travis, T. A., & Robbs, R.S. (1993). Effects of examinee gender, standardized-patient gender, and their interaction on standardized patients' ratings of examinees' interpersonal and communication skills. *Academic Medicine, 68*(2), 153-157.

Colliver, J. A., Marcy, M. L., Travis, T. A., & Robbs, R. S. (1991). The interaction of student gender and standardized-patient gender on a performance-based examination of clinical competence. *Academic Medicine, 66*(9 Suppl), S31-33.

Colliver, J. A., Swartz, M. H., & Robbs, R. S. (2001). The effect of examinee and patient ethnicity in clinical-skills assessment with standardized patients. *Advances in Health Sciences Education: Theory and Practice, 6*(1), 5-13.

Cooke, M.L. (1910). *Academic and industrial efficiency; a report to the Carnegie foundation for the advancement of teaching.* New York: Carnegie Foundation.

Crouse, J. & Trusheim D. (1988). *The case against the SAT.* Chicago: University of Chicago Press.

Cushieri, A., Gleeson, F. A., Harden, R. M., & Wood, R. A. (1979). A new approach to a final examination in surgery: Use of the objective structured clinical examination. *Annals of the Royal College of Surgeons of England, 61*(5), 400-405.

Cusimano, M. D., Cohen, R., Tucker, W., Murnaghan, J., Kodama, R., & Reznick, R. (1994). A comparative analysis of the costs of administration of an OSCE. *Academic Medicine, 69*(7), 571-576.

Dauphinee, D. (2004). Evaluation and the Royal College of Physicians and Surgeons of Canada: A 35-year story of initiatives and influence. In H. B. Dinsdale & G. Hurteau (Eds.), *The evolution of specialty medicine: 1979-2004* (pp. 109-143). Ottawa: Royal College of Physicians and Surgeons of Canada.

Davidson, R. G. (1983). A point of view - Oral examinations. *Annals Royal College of Physicians and Surgeons of Canada, 16*, 114.

Davis, M. (2003). OSCE: the Dundee experience. *Medical Teacher, 25*(3), 255-261.

Dehli, K. (2003). 'Making' the parent and the researcher: Genealogy meets ethnography in research on contemporary school reforms. In M. Tamboukou & S. E. Ball (Eds.), *Dangerous encounters: Genealogy and ethnography* (pp. 133-151). New York: Peter Lang Publishers.

Denzin, N. K., & Lincoln, Y. S. (Eds.). (2000). *Handbook of qualitative research, 2nd Ed.* Thousand Oaks, California: Sage Publications.

Dhruvarajan V. (2005). Colonialism and capitalism: Continuities and variations in strategies of domination and oppression. In P. Tripp & L. Muzzin (Eds.), *Teaching as activism: Equity meets environmentalism* (pp. 134-148). Montreal & Kingston: McGill-Queen's University Press.

Dillon, G. F., Boulet, J., Hawkins, R.E., & Swanson, D. B. (2004). Simulations in the United States Medical Licensing Examination (USMLE) *Quality and Safety in Health Care, 13*(Suppl 1), i41-i45.

Dinsdale, H. B., & Hurteau, G. (Eds.). (2004). *The evolution of specialty medicine: 1979-2004.* Ottawa: Royal College of Physicians and Surgeons of Canada.

Dorsey, J.K., & Colliver, J.A. (1995). Effect of anonymous test grading on passing rates as related to gender and race. *Academic Medicine, 70*(4), 321-323.

Dowdle, M. W. (2006). *Public accountability: Designs, dilemmas and experiences.* Cambridge, UK: Cambridge University Press.

Dreyfus, H. L. & Rabinow P. (1982). *Michel Foucault: Beyond structuralism and hermeneutics.* Chicago: University of Chicago Press.

Education Commission on Foreign Medical Graduates (2006). *ECFMG.* Retrieved April 28, 2006, from http://www.ecfmg.org/index.html.

Eisenhower, D. D. (1953). *Atoms for Peace. Address of the President of the United States of America, to the 470th Plenary Meeting of the United Nations General Assembly. Tuesday, 8 December 1953, 2:45 p.m. World Nuclear Association Webpage.* Retrieved November 1, 2006, from http://www.world-nuclear.org/policy/atomsforpeace.htm.

Elman, B. A. (2000). *A cultural history of civil examinations in late imperial China.* Berkeley, California: University of California Press.

Fairclough, N. (1989). *Language and power.* London: Longman.

Fairclough, N. (1995). *Critical discourse analysis: The critical study of language.* New York: Longman.

Fairclough, N. (2003). *Analyzing discourse: Textual analysis for social research.* New York: Routledge.

Field, J. (1970). Medical education in the United States: Late 19th and early 20th centuries. In C.D. O'Malley (Ed.), *The history of medical education.* Berkeley, California: University of California Press.

Flexner, A. (1925). *Medical education: A comparative study.* New York: Macmillan.

Foucault, M. (1972). *The archaeology of knowledge and the discourse on language.* (A. M. Sheridan Smith, Trans.). New York: Pantheon Books. (Original work published in 1969).

Foucault, M. (1980). *Power/knowledge: selected interviews and other writings 1972-1977* (C. Gordon, L. Marshall, J. Mepham, & K. Soper, Trans.; C. Gordon, Ed.). New York: Pantheon Books. (Original works published 1972-1977).

Foucault, M. (1988). *Madness and civilization; A history of insanity in the age of reason.* (R. Howard, Trans.). New York: Vintage Books. (Original work published in 1961).

Foucault, M. (1988). *The care of the self: The history of sexuality (Vol. 3).* (R. Hurley, Trans.). New York: Vintage books. (Original work published in 1984).

Foucault, M. (1990). *The history of sexuality: An introduction (Vol. 1).* (R. Hurley, Trans.). New York: Vintage Books. (Original work published in 1976).

Foucault, M. (1990). *The use of pleasure: The history of sexuality (Vol. 2).* (R. Hurley, Trans). New York: Vintage Books. (Original work published in 1984).

Foucault, M. (1991). 'Governmentality,' Ideology and Consciousness 6, pp. 5-21. Reprinted in Burchell, G., Gordon, C., and Miller, P. (Eds.) *The Foucault effect: Studies in governmentality.* Chicago: The University of Chicago Press. (Original work published in 1979).

Foucault, M. (1994). Genealogy and social criticism. In Steven Seidman (Ed.) *The postmodern turn: New perspectives on social theory* (pp. 39-45). Cambridge, Mass. Cambridge University Press. (Original work published 1972-1977).

Foucault, M. (1995). *Discipline and punish: The birth of the prison.* (A. M. Sheridan, Trans.). New York: Vintage Books. (Original work published in 1975).

Foucault, M. (1997). *Ethics subjectivity and truth.* (R. Hurley et al, Trans.; P. Rabinow, Ed.). New York: The New Press.

Foucault, M. (1998). On the Ways of Writing History. (R. Hurley, Trans.). (Original work published in 1967). In J. Faubon (Ed.), *Aesthetics, method, and epistemology: Essential works of Foucault (Vol. 2)* (pp. 279-297). New York: The New Press.

Foucault, M. (1998). Return to History. (R. Hurley, Trans.) (Original work published in 1972). In J. Faubon (Ed.), *Aesthetics, method, and epistemology: Essential works of Foucault (Vol. 2)* (pp. 419-432). New York: The New Press.

Foucault, M. (2002). *The order of things.* (Tavistock/Routledge, Trans.). London: Routledge Classics. (Original work published in 1966).

Foucault, M. (2003). *The birth of the clinic.* (A. M. Sheridan, Trans.). London: Routledge. (Original work published 1963).

Fox, R. (1989). *The sociology of medicine.* Englewood Cliffs, NJ: Prentice Hall.

Franke, W. (1960). *The reform and abolition of the traditional Chinese examination system.* Cambridge, Mass: Harvard University Press.

Friedson, E. (1970). *Profession of Medicine.* New York: Harper and Row.

Friedman, M., Sutnick, A. I., Stillman, P. L., Norcini, J. J., Anderson, S. M., Williams, R. G., et al. (1991). The use of standardized patients to evaluate the spoken-English proficiency of foreign medical graduates. *Academic Medicine, 66*(9 Suppl), S61-S63.

Furman, G., Colliver, J. A., & Galofre, A. (1993). Effects of student gender and standardized-patient gender in a single case using a male and a female standardized patient. *Academic Medicine, 68*(4), 301-303.

General Medical Council. (1993). *Tomorrow's doctors: Recommendations on undergraduate medical education.* London: General Medical Council.

Gidney, R., & Millar, W. (1994). *Professional gentlemen. The professions in nineteenth century Ontario.* Toronto: University of Toronto Press.

Gieryn, T. F. (1983). Boundary work and the demarcation of science from non-science: Strains and interests in professional ideologies of scientists, *American Sociological Review, 48*(6), 781-795.

Godkins, T. R., Duffy, D., Greenwood, J., & Stanhope, W. D. (1974). Utilization of simulated patients to teach the 'routine' pelvic examination. *Journal of Medical Education, 49,* 1174-1178.

Goffman, E. (1959). *The presentation of self in everyday life.* London and New York: Doubleday.

Gonnella, J. S. (1979). Evaluation of competence, performance, and health care. *Journal of Medical Education, 54*(10), 825-827.

Gould, S. J. (1981). *The Mismeasure of Man.* New York: WW Norton and Company.

Govaerts, M. J., van der Vleuten, C. P., Schuwirth, L. W. (2002). Optimising the reproducibility of a performance-based assessment test in midwifery education. *Advances in Health Sciences Education: Theory and Practice, 7*(2), 133-145.

Grand'Maison, P., Brailovsky, C. A., Lescop, J., & Rainsberry, P. (1997). Using standardized patients in licensing/certification examinations: Comparison of two tests in Canada. *Family Medicine, 29*(1), 27-32.

Grand'Maison, P., Lescop, J., Rainsberry, P., & Brailovsky, C. A. (1992). Large-scale use of an objective, structured clinical examination for licensing family physicians. *Canadian Medical Association Journal, 146*(10), 1735-1740.

Grand'Maison, P., Brailovsky, C., & Lescop, J. (1997). The Quebec objective structured clinical examination: Modifications and improvements over 6 years of experience. In A. J. J. A. Scherpbier, C. P. M. van der Vleuten, J. J. Rethans, A. F. W. van der Steig (Eds.), *Advances in Medical Education* (pp. 437-440). Dordrecht: Kluver Academic Publishers.

Gutting, G. (1989). *Michel Foucault's Archaeology of Scientific Reason.* Cambridge, UK: Cambridge University Press.

Hafferty, F. W., McKinlay, J. B. (Eds.). (1993). *The changing medical profession: An international perspective.* New York: Oxford University Press.

Hanna, M., Fins. J. J. (2006). Why simulation training ought to be complemented by experiential and humanist learning. *Academic Medicine. 81*(3), 265-270.

Hanson, F. A. (1993). *Testing testing: Social consequences of the examined life.* Berkeley, California: University of California Press.

Harden, R. M., Stevenson, M., Downie, W. W., & Wilson, G.M. (1975). Assessment of clinical competence using objective structured examination. *British Medical Journal, 1*(5955), 447-451.

Harden, R. M., Gleason, F. A. (1979). Assessment of clinical competence using an objective structured clinical examination. *Medical Education, 13*(1), 41-47.

Haraway, D. J. (1988). Situated knowledges: The science question in feminism and the privilege of partial perspective. *Feminist Studies, 14*, 575-599.

Harris, I. B., & Simpson, D. (2005). Christine McGuire: At the heart of the maverick measurement maven. *Advances in Health Sciences Education: Theory and Practice 10*(1), 65-80.

Hartman, H. (1979). Capitalism, patriarchy and job segregation by sex. In Eisenstein Z. R. (Ed.), *Capitalist patriarchy and the case of socialist feminism* (pp. 206-247). New York: Monthly Review Press.

Hartog, P. J. (1918). *Examinations and their relation to culture and efficiency.* London: Constable and Company.

Heins, M., Stillman, P., Sabers, D., & Mazzeo, J. (1983). Attitudes of pediatricians toward maternal employment. *Pediatrics, 72*(3), 283-90.

Hodges, B. (2003a). OSCE! Variations on a theme by Harden. *Medical Education, 37*(12), 1134-1140.

Hodges, B. (2003b). Validity and the OSCE. *Medical Teacher, 25*(3), 250-254.

Hodges, B. (2004). Medical student bodies and the pedagogy of self-reflection, self-assessment and self-regulation. *Journal of Curriculum Theorizing, 20*(2), 41-51.

Hodges, B. (2005). The many and conflicting histories of medical education in Canada and the United States: An introduction to the paradigm wars. *Medical Education, 39*(6), 613-621).

Hodges, B., & Herold-McIlroy, J. (2003). Analytic OSCE global ratings are sensitive to level of training. *Medical Education, 37*(11), 1012-1016.

Hodges, B., & Lofchy, J. (1997). Examining psychiatry clinical clerks with a mini-OSCE. *Academic Psychiatry, 21*(4), 219-225.

Hodges, B., Regehr, G., Hanson, M., & McNaughton, N. (1997). Evaluating psychiatric clinical clerks with an objective structured clinical examination. *Academic Medicine, 72*(8), 715-721.

Hodges, B., Regehr, G., Hanson, M., & McNaughton, N. (1998). The objective structured clinical exam in psychiatry: A validation study. *Academic Medicine, 73*(8), 74-76.

Hodges, B., Regehr, G., McNaughton N., Tiberius, R., & Hanson, M. (1999). OSCE checklists do not capture increasing levels of expertise. *Academic Medicine, 74*(10), 64-69.

Hodges, B., Regehr, G., McNaughton, N., Tiberius, R., & Hanson, M. (2002). The challenge of creating OSCE measures to capture the characteristics of expertise. *Medical Education, 36*(8), 742-748.

Hodges, B., Turnbull, J., Cohen, R., Bienenstock, D., & Norman, G. (1996). Evaluating communication skills in the OSCE format: Reliability and generalizability. *Medical Education, 30*(1), 38-43.

Hoskin, K., W. (1993). Education and the genesis of disciplinarity: The unexpected reversal. In E. Messer-Davidow, D.R. Shumway & D.J. Sylvan (Eds.), *Knowledges: Historical and critical studies in disciplinarity.* Charlottesville: University of Virginia Press.

Howley, L. D. (2004). Performance assessment in medicine: Where we've been and where we're going. *Evaluation and the Health Professions, 27*(3), 285-303.

Hoy, D. C. (1986). *Foucault: A critical reader.* New York: Basil Blackwell.

Hunter, I. (1996). Assembling the School. In A. Barry, T. Osborne & N. Rose (Eds.), *Foucault and political reason: Liberalism, neo-liberalism and rationalities of government* (pp. 143-166). Chicago: University of Chicago Press.

Jayawickramarajah, P. T. (1985). Oral examinations in medical education. *Medical Education, 19*(4), 290-293.

Johnson, T. (1972). *Professions and Power.* London: Routledge.

Kendall, G., & Wickham, G. (2003). *Using Foucault's methods.* London: Sage Publications.

Kohler, C., Braun, M., Mari, G., & Roland, J. (2003). Évolution du profil des étudiants ayant passé le concours de PCEM1 à la Faculté de Médecine de Nancy de 1992 à 2001. *Pédagogie Médicale, 4*(1), 12-17.

Kowlovitz, V., Hoole, A. J., & Sloane, P. D. (1991). Implementing the objective structured clinical examination in a traditional medical school. *Academic Medicine, 66*(6), 345-347.

Kvale, S. (1996). *InterViews: An introduction to qualitative research interviewing.* Thousand Oaks, California: Sage Publications.

Kwolek-Folland, A. (1994). *Engendering business: Men and women in the corporate office.* Baltimore: Johns Hopkins University Press.

Lai, T. C. (1970). *A Scholar in Imperial China.* Hong Kong: Kelly and Walsh.

Langley, D. G. (1994). Certification in psychiatry and neurology: Past, present and future. In J. H. Shore & S. C. Scheiber (Eds.), *Certification, recertification and lifetime learning in psychiatry* (pp. 19-34). Washington, DC: American Psychiatric Press.

Larkin, G. (1983). *Occupational Monopoly and Modern Medicine.* London: Tavistock

Larson, M. (1977). *The rise of professionalism: A sociological analysis.* Berkeley, California: University of California Press.

Larson, M. (1980). Proletarianization and educated labour. *Theory and Society, 9*(1), 131-177.

Light, D. (1993). Countervailing power: The changing character of the medical profession in the United States. In F. W. Hafferty & J. B. McKinlay (Eds.), *The changing medical profession: An international perspective* (pp. 69-80). New York: Oxford University Press.

Livingstone, R. A., & Ostrow, D. N. (1978). Professional patient-instructors in the teaching of the pelvic examination. *American Journal of Obstetrics and Gynecology, 132*(1), 64-67.

Lloyd, J. S. (Ed.). (1982). *Evaluation of non-cognitive skills and clinical performance.* Chicago: American Board of Medical Specialties.

Ludmerer, K. M. (1985). *Learning to heal.* New York: Basic Books.

MacLeod, R. (1982). *Days of judgment: Science, examinations and the organization of knowledge in later Victorian England.* North Humberside, UK: Nafferton Books.

Magnusson, J. (2000). Canadian higher education and citizenship in the context of state restructuring and globalization. *Encounters on Education,* 1(Fall), 107-123.

Major, D. A. (2005). OSCEs: Seven years on the bandwagon: The progress of an objective structured clinical evaluation programme. *Nurse Education Today, 25*(6), 442-454.

Mankin, H. (1981). Oral examination techniques in the non-cognitive domains. In J. S. Lloyd (Ed.) *Evaluation of non-cognitive skills and clinical performance* (pp. 25-31). Chicago: American Board of Medical Specialties.

Manogue, M., & Brown, G. (1998). Developing and implementing an OSCE in dentistry. *European Journal of Dental Education, 2*(2), 51-57.

Matsell, D. G., Wolfish, N. M., & Hsu, E. (1991). Reliability and validity of the objective structured clinical examination in paediatrics, *Medical Education, 25*(4), 293-299.

McFaul, P.B., Taylor, D.J., & Howie, P.W. (1993). The assessment of clinical competence in obstetrics and gynecology in two medical schools by an objective structured clinical examination, *British Journal of Obstetrics and Gynaecology, 100*(9), 842-846.

McGuire, C. (1966). The oral examination as a measure of professional competence. *Journal of Medical Education, 41,* 267-274.

McGuire, C. (1994). Fundamental issues in certification and recertification. In J. H. Shore & S. C. Scheiber (Eds.), *Certification, recertification and lifetime learning in psychiatry* (pp. 35-48). Washington, DC: American Psychiatric Press.

McNaughton, N., Tiberius, R., & Hodges B. (1999). Effects of portraying psychologically and emotionally complex standardized patient roles. *Teaching and Learning in Medicine 11*(3), 135-141.

Medical Council of Canada (2006). *Medical Council of Canada News.* Retrieved April 28, 2006, from http://www.mcc.ca/english/news/index.html.

Miller, G. (1990). The assessment of clinical skills/competence/performance. *Academic Medicine, 65*(9), S63-S67.

Montgomery, R. J. (1965). *Examinations: An account of their evolution as administrative devices in England.* London: Longmans, Green & Co.

Morris, N. (1961). An historian's view of examinations. In S. Wiseman (Ed.), (1961). *Examinations and English education*. Manchester: Manchester University Press.

Mullins, L. (1999). *Management and Organizational Behaviour, 5th Ed*. London: Pitman Publishing.

Muzzin, L. (2005). The brave new world of professional education. In P. Tripp & L. Muzzin (Eds.), *Teaching as activism: Equity meets environmentalism* (pp. 149-166). Montreal & Kingston: McGill-Queen's University Press.

Muzzin, L. J., & Hart, L. (1985). Oral examinations. In V. R. Neufeld & G. R. Norman (Eds.), *Assessing clinical competence* (pp. 71-94). New York: Springer Publishing Company.

Nayer, M. (1993). An overview of the objective structured clinical examination. *Physiotherapy Canada, 45*(3), 171-178.

Nelson, S., & Purkis, M.E. (2004). Mandatory reflection: the Canadian reconstitution of the competence nurse. *Nursing Inquiry*, 11(4):247-257.

Neufeld, V. R., & Norman, G. R. (1985). *Assessing Clinical Competence*. New York: Springer Publishing Company.

Norman, G. (2005a). Editorial--checklists vs. ratings, the illusion of objectivity, the demise of skills and the debasement of evidence. *Advances in Health Sciences Education: Theory and Practice, 10*(1), 1-3.

Norman, G. (2005b). What makes a good doctor? Keynote plenary presentation, Association for Medical Education in Europe Annual Conference, Amsterdam.

Norman, G. R., Neufeld, V. R., Walsh, A. W., Woodward, C. A., & McConvey, G.A. (1985). Measuring physicians' performances by using simulated patients. *Journal of Medical Education, 60*(12), 925-934.

Norwood, W. F. (1970). Medical education in the United States before 1900. In C.D. O'Malley (Ed.), *The history of medical education*. Berkeley, California: University of California Press.

Nunnaly, J. (1978). *Psychometric theory*. New York: McGraw-Hill.

O'Malley, C.D. (1970). *The history of medical education*. Berkeley, California: University of California Press.

O'Malley, P., Weir, L. & Shearing, C. (1997). Governmentality, criticism, politics. *Economy and society*. (26(4): 501-517.

Owen, A., & Winkler, R. (1974). General practitioners and psychosocial problems: An evaluation using pseudo patients. *Medical Journal of Australia, 2*, 393-398.

Pecheux, M. (1975). *Language, semantics and ideology*. New York: St. Martin's Press.

Pinel, P. (1802). *La médecine clinique*. Paris.

Poenaru D., Morales D., Richards A., & O'Connor H.M. (1997). Running an objective structured clinical examination on a shoestring budget. *American Journal of Surgery, 177*(6), 538-541.

Popkewitz, T.S. & Brennan, M. (1998). Foucault's challenge: discourse, knowledge, and power in education. New York: Teachers College Press.

Rashdall, H., (1936). The universities of Europe in the Middle Ages. Oxford: Clarendon Press.

Readings, B. (1996). *The university in ruins*. Cambridge, Mass: Harvard University Press.

Reznick, R., Smee, S., Rothman, A., Chalmers, A., Swanson, D., Dufresne, L., et al. (1992). An objective structured clinical examination for the licentiate: Report of the pilot project of the Medical Council of Canada. *Academic Medicine, 67*(8), 487-494.

Reznick, R. K., Smee, S., Baumber, J. S., Cohen, R., Rothman, A., Blackmore, D., et al. (1993). Guidelines for estimating the real cost of an Objective Structured Clinical Examination. *Academic Medicine, 68*(7), 513-517.

Roach, J. (1961). *Public Examinations in England, 1850-1900*. Cambridge, UK: Cambridge University Press.

Rogers, R., Malancharuvil-Berkes, E., Mosley, M., Hui, D., & O'Garro, J. G. (2005). Critical discourse analysis in education: A review of the literature. *Review of Educational Research, 75*(3), 365-416.

Roma, J. & Oriol, A. (2005). Tributes to Miriam. *Medical Teacher, 27*(3), 242-245.

Rose N. (1996). Governing 'advanced' liberal democracies. In Osbourne, B. & Rose, N. (Eds.) *Foucault and political reason*. Chicago: University of Chicago Press.

Rose, N.S. (1985). *The psychological complex: psychology, politics and society in England, 1869-1939*. London: Routledge.

Rothman, A. & Cohen, R. (1995). Understanding the objective structured clinical examination (OSCE): issues and options. Annals RCPSC

Rowntree, D. (1987). *Assessing students: How shall we know them?* London: Kogan Page.

Royal College of Physicians and Surgeons of Canada (2006). The Royal College of Physicians and Surgeons of Canada. Retrieved April 28, 2006, from http://rcpsc.medical.org.

Sanson-Fisher, R.W. & Poole, A. D. (1980). Simulated patients and the assessment of medical students' interpersonal skills. *Medical Education, 14*(4), 249-253.

Santos, J. & Reynaldo, A. (1999). Cronbach's Alpha: A Tool for Assessing the Reliability of Scales. *Journal of Extension 37*(2). Retrieved December 15, 2005 from http://joe.org/joe/1999april/tt3.html.

Sauer, J., Hodges, B., Santhouse, A. & Blackwood, N. (2004). The OSCE has landed: one small step for British psychiatry? *Academic Psychiatry,* (in press).

Sawicki, J. (1991). *Disciplining Foucault: Feminism, power, and the body*. London: Routledge.

Schermerhorn, J. R. Jr. (1993). *Management for Productivity: Management mistakes and successes*. New York: John Wiley & Sons.

257

Schostak, J.F. (2002). *Understanding, designing and conducting qualitative research in education: Framing the project.* Philadelphia: Open University Press.

Schurwirth, L. W. T. & van der Vleuten, C. P. M. (2006). A plea for new psychometric models in educational assessment. *Medical Education, 40*(4), 296-300.

Segouin, C. & Berard, A. (2005). Principles of a program of quality assurance and evaluation of professional practices. *La Revue du Praticien, 55*(5), 557-564.

Segouin, C. & Hodges, B. (2005). Educating Physicians in France and Canada: Are the differences based on evidence or history? *Medical Education, 39*(12), 1205-1212.

Segouin, C., Hodges, B., & Brechat, P. H. (2005). Globalization in health care: Is international standardization of quality a step toward outsourcing? *International Journal for Quality in Health Care, 17*(4), 277-279.

Schon, D. A. (1987). *Educating the reflective practitioner: Toward a new design for teaching and learning in the professions.* San Francisco: Jossey-Bass.

Shore, J. H., & Scheiber, S. C. (Eds.). (1994). *Certification, recertification and lifetime learning in psychiatry.* Washington, DC: American Psychiatric Press.

Shorter, E. (1985). *Doctors and their patients: A social history.* New York: Simon and Schuster.

Sibbald D., & Regehr G. (2003). Impact on the psychometric properties of a pharmacy OSCE: Using 1st-year students as standardized patients. *Teaching and Learning in Medicine, 15*(3), 180-185.

Sloan, D. A., Donnelly, M.B., Johnson, S.B., Schwartz, R.W., & Strodel, W.E. (1993). Use of an objective structured clinical examination to measure improvement in clinical competence during the surgical internship, *Surgery, 114*(2) 343-351.

Simpson, M. A. (1976). Medical student evaluation in the absence of examinations. *Medical Education, 10*(1), 22-26.

Skinner, B. F. (1953). *Science and human behavior.* New York: Simon and Schuster.

Smallwood, M.L. (1969). An historical study of examinations and grading systems in early American universities; a critical study of the original records of Harvard, William and Mary, Yale, Mount Holyoke, and Michigan from their founding to 1900. Cambridge: Harvard University Press. (Original work published in 1935).

Smith, D. (2004). Writing the social: Critique, theory and investigations. Toronto: University of Toronto Press.

Sosnoski, J.J. (1993). Examining exams. In E. Messer-Davidow, D.R. Shumway & D.J. Sylvan (Eds.), *Knowledges: Historical and critical studies in disciplinarity.* Charlottesville: University of Virginia Press.

Starr, P. (1982). *The social transformation of American medicine: The rise of a sovereign profession and the making of a vast industry.* United States: Basic Books.

Statistical Package for the Social Sciences (2006). *SPSS.* Retrieved April 28, 2006, from http://www.spss.com/.

Stern, D. T, Friedman Ben-David, M., Norcini, J., Wojtczak, A., & Schwarz, M. R. (2006). Setting school-level outcome standards. *Medical Education, 40*(2), 166-172.

Stern, D. T., Friedman Ben-David, M., De Champlain, A., Hodges, B., Wojtczak, A. & Schwarz, R. (2005). Ensuring global standards for medical graduates: A pilot study of international standard-setting. *Medical Teacher.* 27(3):207-13.

Stillman, P. L. (1984). Expanding the role of non-physician teachers and evaluators. *Journal of the American Medical Women's Association, 39*(2), 54-56.

Stillman, P. L., Burpeau-Di Gregorio, M. Y., Nicholson, G. I., Sabers, D. L., & Stillman, A. E. (1983). Six years of experience using patient instructors to teach interviewing skills. *Journal Medical Education, 58*(12), 941-946.

Stillman, P. L., Haley, H. L., Sutnick, A. I., Philbin, M. M., Smith, S. R., O'Donnell, J., et al. (1991). Is test security an issue in a multi-station clinical assessment? A preliminary study. *Academic Medicine, 66*(9), S25-S27.

Stillman, P L., Levinson, D., Navin, H., & Ruggill, J. S. (1978). Collaborative teaching efforts between a medical and nursing college. *Arizona Medicine, 35*(11), 740-2.

Stillman, P. L., Levinson, D., Ruggill, J., & Sabers, D. (1977). The nurse practitioner as a teacher of physical examination skills. *Annual Conference on Research in Medical Education, 16*, 57-62.

Stillman, P. L., Madigan, H. S., Thompson, D. K., Swanson, D. B., Julian, E., Regan, M. B., et al. (1989). The Medical Education Evaluation Program of the state of Ohio. *Academic Medicine, 64*(8), 454-7.

Stillman P. L., Regan, M. B., Philbin, M., & Haley, H. L. (1990). Results of a survey on the use of standardized patients to teach and evaluate clinical skills. *Academic Medicine, 65*(5), 288-292.

Stillman, P. L., Ruggill, J. S, Rutala, P. J, & Sabers, D. L. (1979). A comparison of physicians and nurse practitioners as instructors in a physical diagnosis course. *Medical Education, 54*(9), 733-734.

Stillman, P. L., Ruggill, J. S., Rutala, P. J., & Sabers, D. L. (1980). Patient instructors as teachers and evaluators. *Medical Education, 55*(3), 186-193.

Stillman, P. L., Ruggill, J.S., & Sabers, D.L. (1978). The use of live models in the teaching of gross anatomy. *Medical Education, 12*(2), 114-116.

Stillman, P. L., Sabers, D. L., & Redfield, D.L. (1976). The use of paraprofessionals to teach interviewing skills. *Pediatrics, 57*(5), 769-774.

Stillman, P L., Sabers, D. L., & Redfield, D. L. (1977). Use of trained mothers to teach interviewing skills to first-year medical students: a follow-up study. *Pediatrics, 60*(2), 165-169.

Stillman, P. L., & Swanson, D. B. (1987). Ensuring the clinical competence of medical school graduates through standardized patients. *Archives of Internal Medicine, 147*(6), 1049-1052.

Stillman, P. L., Swanson, D. B., Smee, S., Stillman, A. E., Ebert, T. H., Emmel, V. S., et al. (1986). Assessing clinical skills of residents with standardized patients. *Annals of Internal Medicine, 105*(5), 762-771.

Stokes, J.F. (1973). *The clinical examination.* Dundee, Scotland: Association for the Study of Medical Education.

Strong-Boag, V. (1981). Canada's women doctors: Feminism constrained. In S. E. D. Shortt (Ed.), *Medicine in Canadian society: Historical perspectives* (pp. 109-129). Montreal & Kingston: McGill-Queen's University Press.

Sutnick, A. I., Stillman P. L., Norcini, J. J., Friedman, M., Regan ,M. B., Williams, R. G., et al. (1993). Educational Commission for Foreign Medical Graduates assessment of clinical competence of graduates of foreign medical schools. *Journal of American Medical Association, 270*(9), 1041-1045.

Sutnick, A. I., Stillman, P. L., Norcini, J. J., Friedman, M., Williams, R. G., Trace, D. A., et al. (1994). Pilot study of the use of the Educational Commission for Foreign Medical Graduates clinical competence assessment to provide profiles of clinical competencies of graduates of foreign medical schools for residency directors. *Academic Medicine, 69*(1), 65-67.

Swanson, D. B. & Stillman, P. L. (1990). Use of standardized patients for teaching and assessing clinical skills. *Evaluation and the Health Professions, 13*(1), 79-103.

Swartz, M. H., Colliver, J. A., & Robbs, R. S. (2001). The interaction of examinee's ethnicity and standardized patient's ethnicity: an extended analysis. *Academic Medicine, 76*(10 Suppl), S96-S98.

Tamblyn, R. M., Abrahamowicz, M. Brailovsky, C., Grand'Maison, P., Lescop, J., Norcini, J., et al. (1998). Association between licensing examination scores and resource use and quality of care in primary care practice. *Journal of the American Medical Association, 280*(11), 989-996.

Tamblyn, R. M., Klass, D. K., Schnabel, G. K., & Kopelow, M. L. (1990). Factors associated with accuracy of standardized patient presentation. *Academic Medicine, 65*(9 Suppl.), S55-S66.

Taylor, F. W. (1911). *The Principles of Scientific Management.* New York: Harper.

Teeple, G. (2000). Globalization and the decline of social reform: into the twenty-first century. Aurora, Ontario: Garamond Press; Amherst, N.Y.: Humanity Books.

Thorndike, E. L. (1922). Measurement in Education. In G. M. Whipple, (Ed.), *Intelligence tests and their uses* (pp. 1-9). Bloomington, Ill: National Society for the Study of Education, Public School Publishing Company.

Torfing, J. (1999). *New theories of discourse: Laclau, Mouffe and Zizek.* Oxford: Blackwell.

Usher, R., & Edwards, R. (1994). *Postmodernism and education: Different voices, different world.* New York: Routledge.

Valberg, L. S., & Stuart, R. K. (1983). A point of view: University in-training evaluation and oral examinations in internal medicine. *Annals of the Royal College of Physicians and Surgeons of Canada, 16*, 513-515.

van der Vleuten, C. P. M. (2000a). Validity of final examinations in undergraduate medical training. *British Medical Journal, 321*(1), 1217-1219.

van der Vleuten, C. P. M., & Swanson, D. (1990). Assessment of clinical skills with standardized patients: State of the art. *Teaching and Learning in Medicine, 2*(2), 58-76.

van Zanten, M., Boulet, J.R., McKinley, D.W. (2004) The influence of ethnicity on patient satisfaction in a standardized patient assessment. *Academic Medicine* 79(10 Suppl):S15-7.

Wallace, P. (1997). Following the threads of an innovation: The history of standardized patients in medical education. *Caduceus, 13*(2), 5-28.

Whelan, G. P., Boulet, J. R., McKinley, D. W., Norcini, J. J., van Zanten, M., Hambleton, R. K., et al. (2005). Scoring standardized patient examinations: Lessons learned from the development and administration of the ECFMG Clinical Skills Assessment (CSA), *Medical Teacher, 27*(3), 200-206.

Wilkinson, T. J., Frampton, C.M., Thompson-Fawcett, M. & Egan, T. (2003). Objectivity in objective structured clinical examinations: Checklists are no substitute for examiner commitment. *Academic Medicine, 78*(2), 219-223.

Windrim, R., Thomas, J., Rittenberg, D., Bodley, J., Allen. V., & Byrne N. (2004). Perceived educational benefits of objective structured clinical examination (OSCE) development and implementation by resident learners. *Journal of Obstetrics and Gynecology of Canada, 26*(9), 815-818.

Wilson, G.M., Lever, R., Harden, R.M., Robertson, J.I. (1969). Examination of clinical examiners. *Lancet,* 1(7584):37-40.

Wittgenstein, L. (1953). *Philosophical Investigations.* (G. E. M. Anscombe, Trans.). New York: MacMillan.

Witz, A., (1992). *Professions and patriarchy.* London: Macmillan Press.

Wolinksy, F. D., (1993). The professional dominance, deprofessionalization, proletarianization and corporatization perspectives: An overview synthesis. In F. W. Hafferty, & J. B. McKinlay (Eds.), *The changing medical profession: An international perspective* (pp. 11-24). New York: Oxford University Press.

Woodward, C. A. & Gliva-McConvey, G. (1995). The effects of simulating on standardized patients. *Academic Medicine, 70*(5), 418-420.

Woodward, C. A., Neufeld, V. R., Norman, G. R., & Stillman, P. L. (1983). Symposium: Simulated patients in evaluation of medical education and practice. *Proceedings of the Annual Conference on Research in Medical Education 22*, 238-44.

Appendix A: Historical Events, Discontinuities and Thresholds

Date	Country	Development	Reference
Before 256 BC	China	Invention of examinations (Chou Dynasty 1122-256)	Hanson 1993:186 Lai 1970:1
618-907	China	Under Tang Dynasty Chinese develop a formal system of examinations to select members for the Imperial Court	Hanson 1993:186 Lai 1970:1
1000	China	Under Sung dynasty, civil service exams open to nearly all Chinese	Hanson 1993:186 Franke 1960:1-7
1368-1662	China	Under Ming dynasty, Chinese civil service exams take a form that will last until 20th century	Hanson 1993:186 Franke 1970:1-7
Medie val	Europe	Craft guilds regulate advancement of craftsmen through juries that judge their work	Hartog 1918:4
Renais sance	Europe	Universities confirm the mastery of candidates knowledge of texts with oral examination panels	Hartog 1918:4 Hanson 1993:192 Rashdall 1936 3:142
1646	USA	Harvard introduces oral examinations	Hanson 1993:192 Smallwood 1935/1969:8
1702	UK	First documented written examination at Trinity College Cambridge in mathematics	Hanson 1993:192 Morris 1961:30
1762	USA	Yale students refuse to submit to examinations except at graduation	Hanson 1993: 192 Smallwood 1935/1969:8
1800	UK	Oxford introduces written examinations	Hanson 1993:192
1830	UK	Oxford and Cambridge abandoning oral examinations for written tests	Hanson 1993:192
1833	USA	Harvard introduces first written examination in mathematics	Hanson 1993:192
1851	USA	Harvard introduces written entrance examination	Hanson 1993:193
1853	UK/India	UK institutes a competitive examination for the Indian Civil Service	Hanson 1993:195
1865	USA	Yale moves from biennial examinations (introduced in early 1800s) to annual examinations	Hanson 1993:193 Smallwood 1935/1969:8
1870	UK	Most positions in the British Civil Service subject to competitive examinations	Hanson 1993:38, Hartog 1918
1880s	US/UK	Critics in the US and UK develop a 'deep suspicion of written tests, fearing they 'stifle the imagination and creative though'	Hanson 1993:198
1900	USA	Examinations become common as a part of each university course, not just annually	Hanson 1993:193
1900	USA	College Entrance Examination Board created to design and administer standard entrance examinations to member colleges	Hanson 1993:214 Crouse and Trusheim 1988:1 Gould 1981
1901	China	China develops a new education system based on western influence	Hanson 1993:191
1905	China	By edict of the empress dowager, Chinese civil service examination is abolished	Hanson 1993:191 Franke 1960:48-7

1905	France	French education ministry commissions psychologist Alfred Binet to create a test of intelligence	Hanson 1993:208, Gould 1981
1916	USA	Stanford psychologist Lewis Terman modified the test (renamed Stanford-Binet) which remains the model for American IQ testing today	Hanson 1993:209, Gould 1981
1915	USA	Frederick J Kelly (later Dean of Education at University of Kansas) devises the first multiple-choice question	Hanson 1993:211
1917	USA	1.75 million men administered the 'Army Alpha' – a multiple-choice version of the intelligence test	Hanson 1993:211, Gould 1981
1919	USA	Carl Campbell Brigham adapts the Army Alpha intelligence test as a college admissions test – named the Scholastic Aptitude Test (SAT). Remained virtually unchanged until the 1970s	Hanson 1993:215 Crouse and Trusheim 1988:22-25, Gould 1981
1936		Burt first discusses ANOVA and exam marks	Brennan 1997
1947	USA	Educational Testing Service established as a non-profit corporation to take over design and administration of tests from the College Entrance Examination Board	Hanson 1993:216 Crouse and Trusheim 1988:25-27
1950		Guilliksen summarizes methods for estimating reliability including internal consistency (later Cronbach's alpha) – basis of the OSCE reliability and the 'standard' of 0.8	Brennan 1997
1951	USA	Cronbach describes Cronbach's alpha	Brennan 1997
Discontinuity: Objects, statements and subject positions related to *performance* emerge			
1964	USA	Howard Barrows first reports on use of "programmed patients" from California	Barrows and Abramson 1964
1966		McGuire reports that study of NBME Oral examinations have inter-reliability of 0.25	McGuire 1966
1969	USA	NBME discontinues oral examinations for licensure in USA	
1970	Canada	Howard Barrows goes to McMaster University and further develops what he now calls "simulated patients"	Barrows and Abrahamson:446
1973	Canada	Gayle Gliva-McConvey becomes the first non-health professional simulated patient trainer at McMaster University	Interview with Gliva McConvey
1975	UK	Harden first describes an OSCE at Dundee in Scotland	Harden 1975
1976	USA	Paula Stillman first reports using para-professionals, nurses and mothers as "patient instructors" in the classroom in Arizona	Stillman et al. 1976, 1977a/b
1979	UK	Dundee Dept of Surgery holds an OSCE, Harden reports on details of the OSCE, including measurement scales	Cushieri 1979, Harden 1979
1979	Canada	OSCE disseminated by Hart in Canada, after working with Harden in Dundee on sabbatical	Barrows and Abrahamson 1964
Discontinuity: Objects, statements and subject positions related to *psychometrics* emerge			
1981	USA	Conference held at Southern Illinois University sponsored by Josiah Macy Jr. Foundation that recommended major new focus on performance-based assessment and creation of consortia to develop SP assessment methods	Wallace 1997
1983	USA	Robert Brennan publishes Generalizability Theory and offers courses in this method at the American Education Research Associate/National Council on Measurement in Education meetings	Brennan 1983
1984	USA	The Association of American Medical Colleges release the	Ainsworth et al.

		General Professional Education for Physicians (GPEP) report which cites an imperative for development of performance-based assessment	1991
1985	USA	Abrahamson's "The Oral Examination: The case for and against" lays out the psychometric agenda (objectivity, reliability, validity) formulating traditional orals rhetorically as "ritual"	Abrahamson 1985
1985	USA	2nd meeting also sponsored by Macy Foundation involving OSCE demonstrations by Abrahamson, Norman, Stillman, Swanson, Taylor, Williams and Barrows.	Wallace 1997
1989	USA-Canada	70% of 142 medical schools using SPs	Stillman et al 199
1990		Psychometric discourse related to SP examinations becomes complex and common: "The method provides maximum likelihood estimates of ability conditional on item characteristic curves modeled by monotone splines"	Abrahamowicz at al. 1990:S25

Discontinuity: Objects, statements and subject positions related to *production* emerge

1991	Canada	Hunger strike by international medical graduates in British Columbia – government sets up an Internal Medical Graduate program that uses a 13 station OSCE for screening.	Andrew and Bate 2000
1992	Canada	Canadian Consensus Conference (and statement) on the Teaching and Assessment of Communication Skills in Canadian Medical Schools. (sponsored by the Canadian Cancer Society, National Cancer Institute of Canada, Lederle and the Associated Medical Services). Key statement – "Doctor-patient communication is integral to quality care. Research reveals major deficits". Recommendations including requiring SP performance-based assessment for licensure	Canadian Cancer Society 1992: 2
1992	Canada	Grand'Maison et all report first use of OSCE for high stakes licensure examination "The new Quebec Comprehensive Licensing Examination: A breakthrough in licensing process."	Grand'Maison et al. 1992, Brailovsky et al. 1992 :539
1992	Canada	Medical Council of Canada pilots tests a national OSCE	Reznick et al 199
1993	UK	General Medical Council releases report: "Tomorrow's Doctors" calling for assessment of performance-based outcomes	GMC 1993
1994	USA	Education Commission on Foreign Medical Graduates pilot tests an OSCE for all international visa applicants	Sutnick et al 1994
1993	USA-Canada	80% of 142 medical schools using SPs	Anderson et al 1994
1995	Canada	MCC launches national 14 station OSCE for all graduates 18 months after MD completed	Reznick at al 199
1995	Canada	Rothman and Cohen argue need for expert psychometricians to deal with complex and sophisticated OSCE analysis	Rothman and Cohen 1995
1995	Canada	Woodward states that SPs are a "profession"	Woodward 1995
1996	USA	ECFMG adopts an OSCE for all US international graduates	Whelan et al 2005
2004	US	NBME launches national mandatory OSCE for all 25,000 US medical graduates in 5 testing centres: Atlanta, LA, Chicago, Houston and Boston	

Appendix B: Participants, Location, Position and Academic Degree

Participant	Location	Position	Degree(s)	*Ethnographic notes (e.g. on personal power relations*
Howard Barrows	Hamilton, Canada	Previously faculty at University of California, then McMaster University, now retired	MD (Neurology)	
Jack Boulet	Philadelphia, USA	Psychometrician with Education Commission on Foreign Medical Graduates (ECFMG)	PhD	
William Burdick	Philadelphia, USA	Medical Director with ECFMG	MD (Internal Medicine)	
Evelyne Caron	Montreal, Canada	Resident, McGill University, representative of Fédération des Médecins Résidents du Québec	MD, resident Obstetrics and Gynaecology	
Devra Cohen	New York, USA	Director Morchand Centre, Mount Sinai University, New York	MEd	
Gary Cole	Ottawa, Canada	Psychometrician and Director of Education Research and Development Unit, Royal College of Physicians and Surgeons of Canada	PhD	My colleague on Royal College of Physicians and Surgeons of Canada Evaluation Committee (which I chair)
Marjorie Davis	Dundee, Scotland	Professor and Director, Department of Medical Education, University of Dundee	MD (Internal Medicine)	
Irfan Dhalla	Toronto, Canada	Resident at University of Toronto and Executive member of Canadian Association of Interns and Residents	MD, resident in Internal Medicine	
Gayle Gliva-McConvey	East Virginia, USA	Assistant Professor and Director Theresa Thomas Clinical Skills Centre, East Virginia University	BA	
Ronald Harden	Dundee, Scotland	Professor of Medical Education at Dundee University, previous Director of Centre for Medical Education	MD (Internal Medicine)	
Jean Ker	Dundee, Scotland	Director of Clinical Skills Centre, Professor of Medicine, University of Dundee	MD (Family medicine)	
Danny Klass	Toronto, Canada	College of Physicians and Surgeons of Ontario, previously National Board of Medical Examiners (USA)	MD (Internal medicine)	
Danette McKinley	Philadelphia, USA	Psychometrician, ECFMG	PhD (Epidemiology)	
Geoff Norman	Hamilton, Canada	Professor McMaster University, Director of Education Research Unit	PhD (Physics)	My co-author of articles in mid-1990s
Paul Preece	Dundee, Scotland	Emeritus Professor of Surgery, University of Dundee	MD (Surgery)	
Glenn	Toronto,	Professor, Department of Surgery,	PhD (Cognitive	Reports to me as

Regehr	Canada	Associate Director, Wilson Centre for Research in Education, University of Toronto	psychology)	Associate Director of Wilson Centre Research in Education, of whi I am Director
Richard Reznick	Toronto, Canada	Chair, Department of Surgery, University of Toronto, VP (Education) University Health Network, previous Chair of the MCC OSCE Test Committee	MD (Surgery) MEd	I report to him in role as VP of the hospital (Univers Health Network) which the researc centre I direct is located
Anja Robb	Toronto, Canada	Director, Standardized Patient Program, Assistant Professor, University of Toronto Department of Family and Community Medicine	MEd	Reports to me as Standardized Pat Program is financially and physically locate the Wilson Centi for Research in Education. Co-teaching on OSC and SP workshop
Sydney Smee	Ottawa, Canada	Manager of Part 2 Examination, Medical Council of Canada	MA, (PhD in progress)	Colleague in the 1990s when I ser on the Medical Council of Cana OSCE test committee
Paula Stillman	Delaware, USA	CEO, Christiana Care, previously medical educators in New England and Arizona and consultant with ECFMG	MD (Pediatrics), MBA	
Diana Tabak	Toronto, Canada	Associate Director of Standardized Patient Program, Lecturer University of Toronto Department of Family and Community Medicine	MSc (in progress)	Colleague for teaching internationally a OSCEs and SPs, notably in Jordar
Robyn Tamblyn	Montreal, Canada	Professor Department of Epidemiology and Biostatistics, McGill University	PhD (Epidemiology)	
Peggy Wallace	San Diego, USA	Director of Professional Development Centre, University of California at San Diego	PhD	
Gerry Whelan	Philadelphia, USA	Medical Director, ECFMG	MD (Emergency Medicine)	
Robert Wood	Dundee, Scotland	Emeritus Professor of Surgery, University of Dundee	MD (Surgery)	

ACKNOWLEDGEMENTS

There are many individuals who made significant contributions to the success of this book. First and foremost, I am grateful to the 25 participants who generously agreed to be interviewed, despite the "non-anonymous" nature of the study. All spoke frankly and openly in a way that provided an extraordinarily rich set of perspectives. I strived to present their words and ideas with accuracy and thoughtfulness, and hope that I have been respectful, particularly in the most critical sections of the book.

Linda Muzzin guided and supported my work for 6 years. Her patience in nurturing the early seeds of my ideas continued unfailingly through the detailed editing and re-editing of my rather long text. Her insistence on solid argument and critique was always balanced with recognition of the difficult nature of critically examining my own professional work. Her commitment to teaching is an inspiration for me as I pursue my own academic career. Jamie-Lynn Magnusson helped me unlock the riddle of studying my own profession from "the inside". Her encouragement to push into difficult areas and think in new ways has been central to the framing of my research. Kari Dehli showed me the brilliance, but also the limitations of the ideas of Michel Foucault. She put a human face on a body of work that can be intimidating. The theoretical richness of my research results from the foundation of understanding she helped me construct.

Completing such a project while also working in the Faculty of Medicine has been a challenge. I am grateful for the support of Don Wasylenki, Cathy Whiteside, Ivan Silver and Richard Reznick, the Chairs and Deans to whom I report, for their generosity and support over 6 years. At the Wilson Centre for Research in Education, the scientists, fellows and administrative staff were a constant source of encouragement. Glenn Regehr frequently helped to cover my duties when my academic demands were great and Mariana Cadavid supported me in a hundred ways.

Four individuals had a direct hand in the successful completion of this work. Ayelet Kuper was of tremendous assistance with my unruly bibliography. Nancy McNaughton and Tina Martimianakis were always interested in discussing my emerging ideas, reading drafts and providing enthusiastic support that sustained me when my work was the most difficult. Without Tina's technical expertise, there would be no printed version. Finally, my long-time assistant Helen Caraoulanis has been there for me throughout this adventure. Her care and commitment are woven into every page of this work and admired by every participant.

In the personal realm, I am aware of the enormous influence of my parents in this journey. My mother is a gifted teacher and model of life-long learning whose energy and enthusiasm have long inspired me. My father is an admired health professional and prolific reader who first showed me the value of critical thinking. Their wisdom and values form the essence of this thesis. Finally, Robert Paul, who has been with me everyday of the last two and a half decades, knows more than anyone what it means to undertake such an effort. Without his patience and unwavering support it would not have happened.

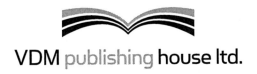
 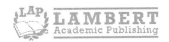 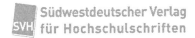